I0766635

Battlefield for Health

Self-Control for a God-Centered Life

By
Cathleen Lerew

BATTLEFIELD FOR HEALTH: SELF-CONTROL FOR A
GOD-CENTERED LIFE

Published by Bodybuilding Potter Publishing.
Biglerville, Pennsylvania
Copyright © 2026 by Cathleen Lerew
All rights reserved.
Printed in the United States of America.
ISBN 979-8-9943101-0-6

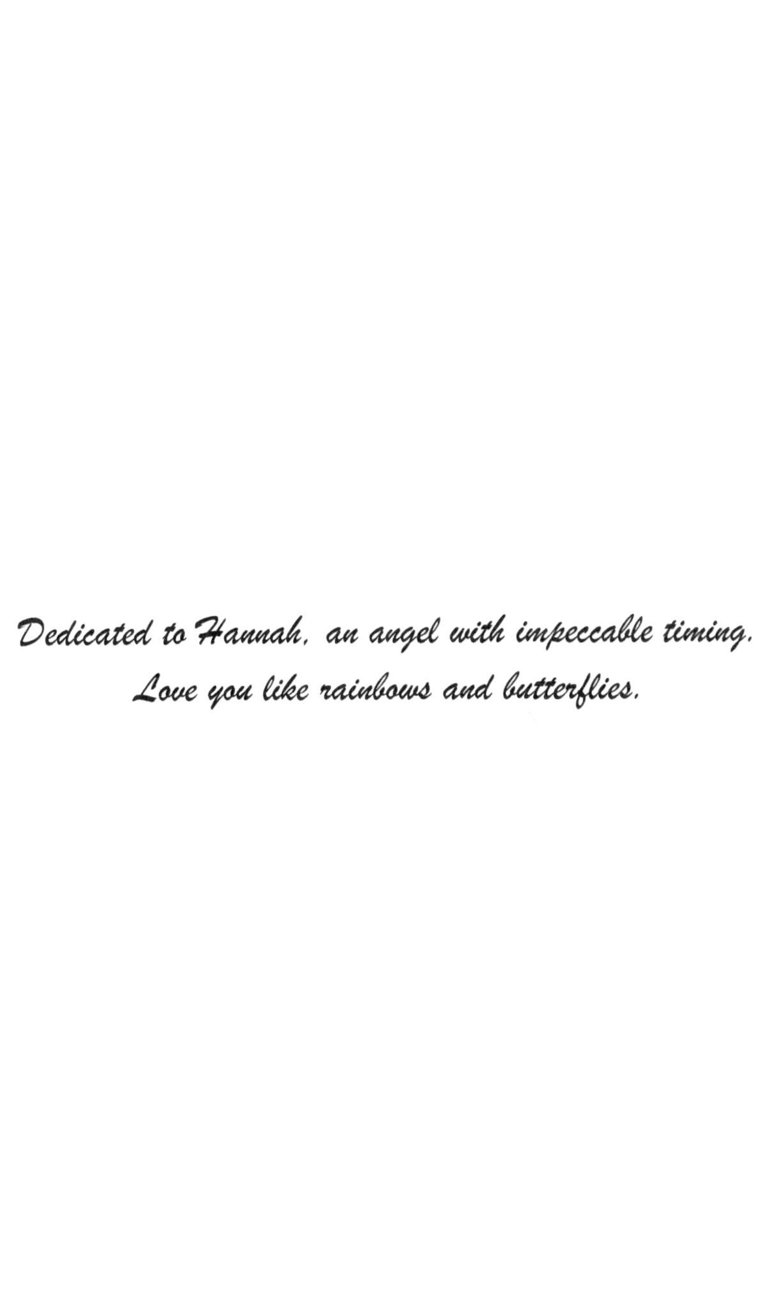

Dedicated to Hannah, an angel with impeccable timing.
Love you like rainbows and butterflies.

Contents

Foreword

By the Author's Daughter, Denae

You didn't pick up this book by accident. Somewhere along the way, something in you knew that the way you've been living striving, pushing, or starting over was no longer sustainable. Maybe you're tired of setting health goals that never last. Maybe you're worn down by caring for everyone else while neglecting yourself. Or maybe you feel stuck, longing for deeper purpose, clarity, and peace. If any of this resonates, take a breath. You are in the right place.

My name is Denae, and I am Coach Cathleen The Bodybuilding Potter's daughter. I've had a front row seat to the story you are about to read. Not the polished version. Not the "after" photo. The real, daily, lived journey of a woman who loved God deeply, yet carried pain - physical, emotional, and spiritual - for far longer than anyone should. I watched my mom show up for everyone around her while quietly battling chronic pain and misdiagnosed postpartum depression for more than 19 years. I saw her pray for healing, try every solution offered, and keep going even when the breakthrough didn't come.

And then, I watched something shift.

What makes this book different, from what I have witnessed firsthand, is that it is not about a quick fix, a rigid program, or a pursuit of perfection. It is about surrender. It is about obedience in small, unglamorous choices. It is about learning to live a God-centered life where faith doesn't sit on the sidelines, but directs every decision, including how we care for our bodies.

I watched my mom turn her health journey over to the Lord completely. Not halfway. Not conditionally. Fully. And in doing so, I saw her become not just a stronger woman, but a healed one.

Her transformation was never just physical. Yes, the outward changes were undeniable, but what impacted me most was the inward work. I saw her confidence return, her joy deepen, and her peace grow steady and rooted. I saw discipline replace chaos, clarity replace overwhelm, and faith replace fear. She didn't become someone new. She became more fully who God had always created her to be.

This book is an extension of that journey.

What you will find in these pages is not theory. It is lived experience. It is a testimony of what happens when faith leads and action follows. My mom doesn't write as someone who has it all figured out, but as someone who has walked the road of trial, surrender, and daily obedience, and continues to walk it.

As her daughter, I can say this with confidence. The principles shared here are real. They work because they are rooted in truth, not trends. They are grounded in Scripture, not shame. And they are offered with grace, not judgment.

This book is an invitation. Not to strive harder, but to trust deeper. Not to control outcomes, but to practice self-control as a fruit of the Spirit. Not to earn worth, but to live from the worth already given to you by God.

If you choose to step into this journey, know that you are not expected to be perfect. You are only asked to be willing. Willing to show up. Willing to surrender. Willing to take one faithful step at a time.

I invite you to let your guard down. Read these words as many times as you need to. Work the pages of this book, not for comparison, not for approval, but for yourself, for your family, and for Him.

I have seen what God can do through a surrendered heart and consistent, faith filled action. My prayer is that, as you turn these pages, you will begin to see what He can do in you as well.

Welcome and Getting Started

Life was never meant to be lived in constant striving, exhaustion, or self-reliance. *Battlefield for Health* invites you to approach life differently—not by doing more, but by living with greater intention. God calls us to glorify Him not only through spiritual moments, but through the way we live our everyday lives—how we eat, move, rest, work, and care for what He has entrusted to us.

In this journey, we will begin by digging—unlearning worldly patterns and renewing our minds with faith-filled truth. From there, we will lay a strong, God-centered foundation, adding bricks one day at a time through small, obedient choices. This is a slow and deeply intentional process of transformation. When even ordinary decisions are offered to God, life becomes less complicated and more purposeful. From this place, a life anchored in faith and built to endure begins to take shape.

You Have Arrived—But Why Are You Here?

- Have you made lots of health goals only to fall short on achieving them?
- Is your life flooded with things to accomplish and/or people to take care of?
- Are your days long with seemingly little time for self-care?

If you answered yes to any of these questions, welcome to the human experience.

- Are you feeling stuck or flat in life?
- Are you desiring a healthier lifestyle?

- Are you desiring a deeper connection and purpose?

If you answered yes to any of these, you are in the right place. And you're not alone. Many of us set out with good intentions, only to find ourselves exhausted, stretched thin, and unsure how to take the next step.

The truth is, lasting change doesn't happen through sheer willpower or the next quick-fix plan—it starts with a strong foundation. Just as a house cannot stand without a solid foundation, your health and life transformation must be built on something unshakable. For me, that foundation is God-centered, anchored in the fruit of the Spirit—self-control.

This is not about striving in your own strength, but exercising self-control by faith in Christ, so that He receives the glory. Through the development of self-control, we exercise our God-given ability to choose to act—or not act—on certain impulses, shaping our daily choices in alignment with His will. With self-control being a fruit of the Spirit (see Galatians 5:22–23), this means we already have this ability! We simply need to learn to exercise it and apply it in our daily lives through surrender and action.

When we approach life with an eager heart to learn, we gain wisdom and knowledge. When we apply that truth, real and lasting transformation begins—strengthening your body, renewing your mind, and deepening your spirit.

This sequence matters: Him → mindset → nourishment → movement. This is how your God-centered healthy lifestyle foundation is dug and your "house" is built on bedrock, not sand.

A Bit About My Journey

My name is Cathleen, and I am the founder of The Body-building Potter. I am excited you are here. As you explore what a God-centered healthy lifestyle looks like for you, it is critically important that you know who I am and where I come from.

The Start of the Official Healing Story

I am…

- A blessed child of God.
- A dedicated and loving wife for over 20 years.
- A blessed momma to 3 amazing young adults and lots of furry babies.
- A dedicated daughter and sister.
- A master potter who sculpts with clay and has had my work in all 50 states and 17 countries. This work gives me a unique perspective on all the mentions in the Bible about the master potter and clay.
- An owner of a successful outreach-based pottery studio.
- Supporter of my husband's professional audio/visual business.
- A natural master's figure bodybuilding competitor who sculpts with fitness and nutrition.
- A black belt in karate.
- A God-centered lifestyle coach.

For 19 years, I lived in some sort of pain—extreme foot and back pain, PCOS, severe postpartum depression, and a deep, lingering depression that shaped every day of my life. Despite all the blessings in my life, and my awareness of them, I often felt ready to give up. I prayed for healing for years and did everything I thought would get me there, yet the breakthrough never came.

Then, in the fall of 2020, God placed a healing journey on my heart. The Holy Spirit's prompting grew more frequent and persistent until I could no longer ignore it. When He told me that, after originally competing in 2002, 21 years later, I would walk on a bodybuilding stage again, I thought, "He must be nuts!" But His message was clear: I would heal by becoming a bodybuilder once more, and I was to glorify Him every step of the way. My prayers for healing—physical and emotional—were answered, but only after I surrendered fully. I had tried my way long enough. So I said, "Yes, Lord." In that moment, more than 160 pounds overweight, I became a bodybuilder again in my heart.

January 2021 marked the official beginning of my healing journey—a journey rooted in God-glorifying self-control and self-discipline. I learned to practice self-control in the smallest daily tasks, which led to greater victories. By quieting the noise of the world, I developed a deeper God-centered lifestyle. The renewal of my mind became the key to my physical transformation. My external change—the one that would carry me to the stage—was simply the reflection of all the work God was doing within me during this season of surrender and movement.

By 2022, my confidence in God's path for me was so strong that I contacted the bodybuilding show promoter from the federation I had competed in back in 2002. I asked about the 2023 show schedule—well over a year in advance. He was understandably surprised, but I knew from past years that the dates were fairly consistent. God had told me to prepare, so I did. I marked September 23, 2023, on my calendar as the day I would step on stage—not just in competition, but in worship.

Over 650 photos now document my journey back to the stage. Since then, I've competed in Pennsylvania, New Jersey, and Texas—even making it to the Summer Shredding Championship and returning to Houston for a second show. Today, I have 7 shows under my belt, each one an opportunity to point to and glorify God.

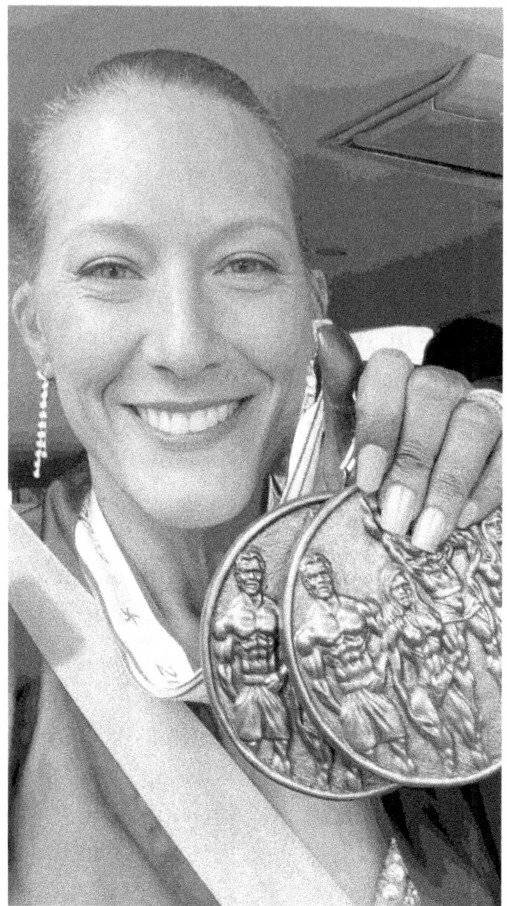

Here's a picture of me at my body-building return in September 2023 with two of my medals.

Somewhere in that process, God impressed on my heart to help others walk their own path of transformation. I had witnessed His miracles firsthand, and my desire to share them became almost uncontainable. I searched for a body-building coach who would lead with faith before fitness and food—but I couldn't find one. While I knew about the sport, I also know the value in education through coaching. My requests were ignored, my convictions misunderstood, and at one point, I was even coached by a wolf in sheep's clothing. In the process, I found a wonderful coach for natural body-building and chose to dig into my faith more on my own through my, now, external transformation.

One day, in a casual conversation with my daughter, I said, "Maybe I'm supposed to be that coach for others." Without hesitation, she replied, "Maybe you should be!" That moment was a turning point. In March 2023, I stepped into the next chapter of my journey—not just as an athlete, but as a coach, called to guide others in their faith-filled, God-centered transformation.

The original program was called Him Centered Coaching. But as the work within our studio (UnderTheHorizon.net) grew, and our outreach expanded, the name evolved. The Bodybuilding Potter became an official division of the studio—and we haven't looked back since.

I'm not a pastor, trainer, or nutritionist. I'm a Christian woman who has experienced God's incredible healing firsthand. I have walked—and continue to walk—a path of surrender and movement, built on self-control, gratitude, faith, and focus through a God-centered lifestyle. I research, learn, and seek tools to glorify God through self-control while achieving the goals He places on my heart. I openly share my healing journey, along with the best practices and habits that have worked for me and my lifestyle.

Having "been there, done that," I understand the struggles and know the tools that can help you build a life anchored in faith and grounded in self-control—a life that brings free-dom, not restriction. My own lifestyle is filled with both "Yes" and "Amen" in my decisions and actions. I learned self-control in the smallest of tasks, and those victories led to the achievement of larger health and fitness goals. By practicing self-control, I was able to quiet the noise of the world and live with a deeper, more God-centered focus.

Truly and deeply, the healthier we are the better we can serve in God's purpose for us and serve others.

Accepting Christ as Your Lord and Savior

Before diving into the daily practices, it is vital to understand one foundational truth: this journey is built on a relationship with Jesus Christ. Accepting Him as your Lord and Savior is the first step, the cornerstone upon which all transformation—spiritual, mental, and physical—can stand.

If you have already accepted Christ as your Lord and Savior, you may choose to skip this section or use it as a time to reaffirm your commitment.

Why Accept Christ?

When you accept Christ, you are inviting forgiveness, restoration, and peace into your life. You are allowing the Holy Spirit to guide, teach, and comfort you. His presence actively leads you, corrects you, encourages you, and brings clarity when the world feels confusing. This is not about knowing all the answers—the beauty of faith is moving forward even when the path is unclear.

Faith is the bridge that allows you to step forward when you don't yet have the full picture. You may not know exactly how every part of this journey will unfold, but choosing to follow Christ ensures your foundation is unshakable. Each act of obedience, each small decision to trust Him, strengthens your walk and aligns your life with His purposes.

How to Accept Christ

Accepting Christ can be simple. It is a step of faith—acknowledging that Jesus is Lord, that He died for your sins, and that you choose to follow Him. A simple prayer might be: *"Lord Jesus, I believe that You are the Son of God. I believe You died for my sins and rose again. I ask You to come into my heart, forgive me, and be my Lord and Savior. Guide my steps, strengthen my faith, and lead me closer to You every day. Amen."*

Saying this prayer with sincerity is the beginning of a personal relationship with Christ. From here, the Holy Spirit begins to work in your life, guiding, strengthening, and comforting you.

A Biblical Example of Faith in Action

Consider Abraham, a man called by God to leave his home and step into the unknown. God did not provide a full roadmap of where Abraham was going. Instead, He called him to take the first step, trusting that God would lead him.

Hebrews 11:8 (AMP): *"By faith Abraham, when he was called [by God], obeyed by going to a place which he was to receive as an inheritance; and he went, not knowing where he was going."*

Like Abraham, your steps of faith today may feel uncertain. You may not see the full path ahead—but as you choose to follow Christ, you are setting a foundation that cannot be shaken.

Program Expectations

This journey is designed to transform your body, mind, and spirit. To gain the most, consider the following expectations:

1. **Give Your Best Every Day**

   Not every day will feel perfect, and not every day will allow you to give 100%. Some days you may wake with only 40% to give, and that is okay. The goal is to give what you have in that moment. At the end of the day, rest knowing you truly gave your best for that day.

2. **Self-Reflection and Honest Communication**
Take time to honestly reflect on your actions, thoughts, and feelings. Journaling, prayer, and quiet reflection will help you identify areas that need growth and those that are thriving. This is a slow, deliberate process—there is no rush.

3. **Follow at Your Own Pace**
Each day's material is a guide, not a strict schedule. Some days you may need more time; other days you may move faster. Track your progress as you go, and remember: this journey is about **progress, not perfection**.

4. **Be a Lifelong Student**
Embrace the process of learning and growth. Grace over perfection should guide your journey. Spiritual, physical, and mental growth is step-by-step, and each day's practice builds on the last.

5. **Trust God Through Every Step**
Every choice you make moves you closer or farther from your foundational dig. Even small victories are significant because they reflect obedience and trust. Remember, your transformation is a lifelong process—one that mirrors Christlikeness more each day.

6. **Consistency Over Intensity**
Small, consistent steps create lasting change. You do not need to accomplish everything at once. Focus on building habits, not on perfection.

7. **Surrender and Faith**

Remember that this journey is not about self-reliance but about surrendering to God's plan. Faith and trust in Him guide every action. Even when the path is unclear, He is shaping your transformation.

8. **Expect Resistance**

A faith-filled life is not always easy, but it is always worth it. As you seek God more deeply, you will encounter resistance. This does not mean you are failing—it means you are growing. You are valued, and what is valuable is often challenged. Stay grounded in God's presence and truth. **Just keep going!** Challenges are not meant to defeat you but to deepen your reliance on Him and strengthen your faith.

How to Use This Book

This book is designed as a flexible, God-centered guide to help you integrate faith into your healthiest life, so you can better serve God's purpose for you and serve others. Together, we will dig a God-centered foundation upon which to build your daily life. Here's how to use it:

Days as Playing Cards

Think of each day as a shuffled deck of cards—you can choose which day to start with. The days do not need to be completed in order. Each card or day helps to dig your God-centered foundation. It is recommended to work through a set of days (1-10, 2-20, etc.) in sequence as there is a built-in reflection day, called a Dig Deeper Day, at the end of each section.

Also, I will be using the Amplified Bible (AMP) for any scripture references I cite throughout the text.

Daily Dig and Actions

Each day includes a "dig," which is a reflection or study designed to renew your mind, and an action step to apply the lesson in real life. This could be journaling, creating a piece of art, or completing a physical or spiritual exercise.

Checkpoints for Progress, Not Perfection

As you move through the book, you'll see opportunities to mark off checkpoints. These are not "done stamps," but reminders that you've dug into the soil of growth on that day. Growth in Christ is cumulative—each reflection adds a layer to your foundation. You may, and are encouraged to, revisit prompts or actions as God deepens your understanding.

Review and Reflection Days

Every so often, you'll find a review day built in – called Dig Deeper Day. These are moments to pause, look back, and notice how God has been working through your reflections and actions. Think of them as chances to connect the dots between past insights and present growth.

Integration of Faith and Practice

Every activity, reflection, and challenge in this book is designed to center your heart on God. Spiritual growth is inseparable from your health journey. As you build self-control, discipline, and focus, you simultaneously strengthen your body, mind, and spirit.

Flexible Pacing

Some days may require more time than others. Some day may need multiple sessions. Some topics are intentionally revisted throughout the book. This is YOUR journey. You set the pace. Just keep going - progress is about moving forward, not racing to the finish line.

Life-Long Journey

This book is not about quick fixes or short-term results. It is about creating a life that is God-centered, faith-anchored, and physically vibrant. As we dig the foundation, we begin adding bricks that strengthen your lifelong health and faith journey.

Digging represents unlearning worldly ways and renewing our minds with faith-filled truth. Building—and each brick laid—represents a God-centered foundation that is strong and capable. This is a lifelong journey of repetition and growth. There is no earthly finish line, because we continue building until we go home with our Lord and Savior. This book is simply an aid to help you dig and build.

Personalization and Ownership

Your path will be unique. Not every activity or reflection will resonate equally. Choose what speaks to you, and let God guide which areas of focus are most relevant for your journey.

A Note About This Journey

Lasting change always begins in the mind and heart. Before your body can change, your thinking must be renewed. Before habits can take root, your beliefs must be aligned. Before discipline can be sustained, your foundation must be anchored in Christ.

Many people begin their personal God-centered healthy lifestyle journey by focusing on the outside — the diet, the steps, the gym sessions, the workout plans. But without addressing the internal world first, many circle the same mountain again and again. We try harder, restart often, burn out quickly, or slip back into old stronghold behaviors.

This book is designed to help break that cycle. It is time to stop circling and start digging!

These 86 days guide you into a deeper connection with God so that your mindset is transformed and your foundation is strengthened. When your inner life is aligned with truth, your outer life can finally grow in the right direction — and stay that way. External transformations are "icing on the cake" — a beautiful bonus, not the main goal.

Throughout these pages, you will find encouragement, reflection, spiritual growth, and discussions around many wellness topics. You will not find specific workouts, sets, reps, or detailed exercise instructions. Why? Because this book is designed to support any established fitness routine, not replace one. After all, the best program is one you can stick with.

Whether you have yet to begin a fitness plan, are already following a program, are working with a trainer, enjoy group classes, or prefer to move at home (my personal favorite), this book is designed to deepen your "why," strengthen your mindset, and prepare your heart. It is the internal work that makes the external efforts sustainable.

The same is true for nutrition. This book will not prescribe a meal plan — because transformation begins with God first, not food rules. Properly fueling our body is critical to a healthy lifestyle. It is not about perfection in eating. If losing weight is a goal, there are many approaches. I never pass judgment on the method chosen; after all, this is a deeper dig than just nutrition. However, I personally support a macro-based approach. Overall, a foundation of proper fueling needs to be built so that if the method changes, the knowledge gained is still maintained and can still be used.

This book helps you:
- Build your foundation before building your routine
- Anchor your identity in Christ before anchoring to macros or metrics
- Cultivate sustainable habits that honor God
- Break stronghold patterns instead of repeating them
- Strengthen your heart, mind, and spirit so your body can follow
- Support your current efforts or awaken a new, deeper approach

If you have been circling the same mountain, this is your invitation to do it differently. Start with Him. Start with truth. Start with renewal from the inside out. And then — when you are ready — connect your renewed mindset to structured steps, movement, and nourishment.

It is recommended to grab a paper and pen. Now... let's walk together — one day, one breath, one obedient step at a time.

Launch Prayer

Lord, I place this journey in Your hands. Dig deep within me, renew my mind, and build a strong, God-centered foundation in my life. Help me walk in obedience, trust You in the process, and keep moving forward with faith. May this journey honor You and prepare me to serve Your purpose. In this your son's name I pray. Amen.

Day 1:
A Look Back and Self-Care

_______________ **Completion Date**

Today, we look back at where you began and start strong building foundation habits. This act of reflection helps anchor your growth.

Self-care is essential. It might mean feeding your body properly with movement, hydration, rest, reading, or taking quiet moments with God. Self-care is not selfish. If you can't care for yourself, it becomes difficult—sometimes impossible—to care for others well.

Side note: Everyone's view of a healthy lifestyle is different, and that's okay. My own version of health is a perfect example of something that doesn't look "typical" to the outside world. What matters most isn't fitting a mold—it's finding what genuinely supports your well-being and honors God in the process.

Deeper Reflection

- How have you prioritized your health up to this point? Consider not only your physical health but also your emotional, mental, and spiritual well-being. Are there areas you've consistently nurtured? Are there areas you've neglected?

- Where do you need to actively create space for self-care? Take a moment to reflect on what _you_ can control in your life—your time, your choices, your energy, and your habits. Self-care doesn't have to be a monumental time commitment. Even small, intentional moments—taken consistently—can create powerful, lasting change over time. Focus on what's within your power to change, rather than blaming circumstances or other people. What could it look like to carve out even a few minutes each day or week to invest in your well-being?

• In what ways have you seen your ability to care for others affected—positively or negatively—by how you care for yourself? Think about the relationships in your life—family, friends, colleagues, or even strangers you encounter daily. When you are physically, mentally, and spiritually nourished, how does that show up in your patience, your presence, and your ability to serve? Conversely, when you are depleted, overwhelmed, or neglecting your own needs, how has that impacted your interactions or the energy you bring to others? Reflect honestly on the connection between your self-care and the quality of care, love, and support you are able to give.

• Identify what self-care looks like for *you*—not what the world says it should look like, and not what works for someone else. Include practical actions that fit your life, such as stocking your kitchen with healthy food choices, moving your body, hydrating, or getting adequate rest. Don't forget practices, like prayer walks, Bible journaling, or quiet time, and fellowship activities—times spent connecting with others in uplifting and supportive ways. Write it down so it becomes a clear. At the very base, choose one small change. Reflect on a specific, realistic change you can make today to better care for yourself. Keep it small enough that it feels doable, but meaningful enough to make a difference—like adding an extra glass of water, taking 10 minutes to stretch, or pausing to pray midday.

• Write down both your definition of self-care and your one small change in a visible place—your journal, a sticky note on your mirror, or as a reminder in your phone.

Tip: Set a daily alarm or reminder on your phone to

prompt you to complete your self-care. Over time, these small, intentional actions will become natural habits.

Verse for Study

1 Corinthians 6:19–20 (AMP): *"Do you not know that your body is a temple of the Holy Spirit who is within you, whom you have [received as a gift] from God, and that you are not your own?*

"You were bought with a price [you were actually purchased with the precious blood of Jesus and made His own]. So then, honor and glorify God with your body."

Tool for your journey
Self-Care Daily Check Box Counter –
A practice in obedience not in perfection.

Month: _______________________

Sun	Mon	Tue	Wed	Thu	Fri	Sat
☐	☐	☐	☐	☐	☐	☐
☐	☐	☐	☐	☐	☐	☐
☐	☐	☐	☐	☐	☐	☐
☐	☐	☐	☐	☐	☐	☐
☐	☐	☐	☐	☐	☐	☐

Tip: Put this where you'll see it daily—on your fridge, bathroom mirror, or nightstand—and mark each day you complete your self-care. Over time, watch your streak grow as consistency builds healthy habits.

Day 2:
Receiving God's Love

___________ **Completion Date**

Before you can give love or serve effectively, you must receive God's love.

Think of it like the instructions you hear on an airplane: in an emergency, you're told to put on your own oxygen mask before assisting anyone else. It isn't because you don't care about the people around you—it's because you can't help them if you're gasping for air yourself. The same is true in life: if you're running on empty, your ability to love, serve, and show up for others will be limited. You cannot pour from an empty cup. To receive God's love, you must be open—mindfully, actively, and eagerly.

Deeper Reflection

- What does receiving God's love look like in your life? Consider how you personally experience His love—through prayer, Scripture, worship, time in nature, the encouragement of others, or moments of peace in your heart. Are there specific ways you've seen His love expressed toward you recently? How do you respond to that love in your daily choices and in how you care for yourself? *For me, I begin each morning by simply saying, "Lord, I receive Your love." It's my small effort to give Him my first moments each day, right when my eyes open.*

- When do you feel most open to His presence? Think about the environments, activities, and attitudes that make you most aware of God's nearness. Is it during quiet early mornings, while singing worship, serving others, or even while moving your body in exercise? Reflect on how you can create more space for those moments, so your awareness of His presence becomes a regular part of your rhythm.

There's no checklist here. It's a journey, not a task. But actively recognizing His love changes how you act and serve.

Verse for Study

1 John 4:19 (AMP): *"We love, because He first loved us."*

Tools for Your Journey

Prayer Prompt: "Lord, I receive Your love today. Help me to be rooted and established in it. Let Your love fill me so completely that it overflows into every word I speak, every action I take, and every person I encounter. Remind me that I can only give what I first receive from You. Amen."

Day 3:
Savoring the Journey

__________ Completion Date

Most days, I wake up feeling like I'm living in a dream. My resting heart rate is low, my body is strong, and I move with ease—proof of the work God has done in my life.

It's time to dig in and really prepare our hearts for this next step. Before we begin, I want to start with a prayer of protection—sometimes called a "hedge of protection." I came across one that I think says it perfectly:

"Dear Heavenly Father, thank You for loving me and reminding me of Your truth. Help me to keep my eyes on You, especially in times of rejection. May I remember that You can use all things for my good and for Your glory. Give me a heart that trusts You, and take away the desire to lean on my own understanding. In Your Son's name I pray, Amen."

This journey we're on is deeply personal and deeply different for everyone. I've said before—and I'll say it again—don't compare your pace to anyone else's. You're not behind. You're not too slow. You're not "less than." God designed your journey specifically for you, and walking it out authentically is the key to growth.

I think back to my first full competitive season after returning to bodybuilding. After being healed from years of setbacks, it was a season of stepping fully into who God had made me to be. The preparation wasn't easy—it was years of consistent work, mental focus, but more so daily surrender with movement towards His plan.

I remember one day in particular, pushing past my comfort zone. I had been practicing mandatory poses in the gym. These poses are how bodybuilders present themselves on stage during the show. There was really no space for this activity at the gym even though this was the perfect location (at the time) for this fitness work. In her true form, my daughter encouraged me to take it one step further: "Mom, put your heels on."

These weren't just any heels—they were clear, platform stilettos, an essential part of stage presentation. Walking in them at the gym felt completely foreign, but I reminded myself that preparation is practice for the life we want to live. I put on the heels, stood tall, and moved through my routine, in the very center area of the gym, fully aware that I was exactly where God had placed me. People might have had opinions, but it didn't matter—I was doing what I was called to do.

That season taught me so much. I had what I needed: faith, discipline, and consistency. Not long after, I canceled my gym membership and began working out at home – never looking back. My workout time has become one of my most prayer-filled times of my week.

That's the same for you. You are exactly where God has you right now. Growth, change, and transformation are inevitable, but permanent change requires more than surface-level **effort—it requires a shift in how we think, act, and live.**

The destination is not what matters most. Savor the journey. Every tiny action, every small improvement, counts.

Deeper Reflection

- Identify one small win in your journey today. Take a moment to pause and notice even the smallest victories. Maybe you chose to eat a nourishing meal, moved your body, spent intentional time in prayer, or simply gave yourself grace instead of criticism. Small wins build momentum and reinforce your commitment to living a God-centered, healthy life. Celebrate them—they are proof that progress is happening, even when it feels slow.

- How can you focus on progress rather than perfection? Reflect on the difference between striving for perfection and embracing steady growth. Perfection often leads to discouragement, while focusing on progress helps you see the value in each step forward. What actions, attitudes, or thought patterns can you adopt today to honor effort over flawless execution? How can you remind yourself that consistent small steps, guided by God, are what truly create lasting change?

Verses for Study

John 8:32 (AMP): *"And you will know the Truth [regarding salvation], and the Truth will set you free [from the penalty of sin]."* Facing the truth about ourselves—our habits, our fears, and our excuses—is one of the bravest things we can do. And when we do, God walks with us every step of the way, setting us free to live the life He's called us to.

Matthew 6:34 (AMP): *"So do not worry about tomorrow; for tomorrow will worry about itself. Each day has enough trouble of its own."*

Tools for your journey

Prayer Prompt: "Lord, help me to step boldly into the life You've called me to, even when it feels uncomfortable. Give me the courage to prepare for what's ahead, the humility to face the truth, and the faith to trust Your plan. Amen."

Day 4:
Abide

Jesus gave us the first principle to follow when it comes to winning the battle of the mind. He said that if we abide in His Word—continually obeying it and living in accordance with His teachings—we will know the truth, and the truth will set us free. God's Word is truth. It all starts there.

True freedom comes from receiving God's truth and applying it to every area of our lives through obedience. This is where self-control and self-discipline come in. Freedom does not mean that the challenges, habits, or struggles we face disappear completely. Rather, freedom means that the stronghold in our life has been broken—the controlling power it once had over our thoughts, actions, or emotions is released. We gain wisdom, understanding, and the tools to respond differently, even when difficult situations arise.

A stronghold is anything in our life that has taken a position of authority over our mind or behavior—a belief, habit, fear, or pattern that keeps us trapped in cycles of defeat, distraction, or limitation. Often, the enemy works patiently over years, carefully laying the groundwork so that these strongholds take root. They can feel permanent or unmovable—until God's truth enters the situation. Once His truth is applied, we gain the power and insight to respond differently. Freedom is not about the problem disappearing; it's about the stronghold losing its control and us learning to walk in victory, equipped with God's wisdom.

By drawing on the power of the Holy Spirit, and not on our

own limited abilities, He will always lead you to freedom. That truth has guided me through every step since. Reflecting on my own life, I've seen strongholds in the form of fear, self-doubt, and lingering habits of comparison. The enemy had been patient, subtly trying to convince me that I wasn't ready, capable, or worthy of the next step. Yet, as I leaned into God, trusted His Spirit, and obeyed His Word, I saw those strongholds loosen. I learned to respond differently, step boldly, and walk in freedom—even when challenges remained.

This journey is not a quick fix. It is not about rushing or skipping over the hard parts. Every moment—the triumphs, the struggles, even the tears—has value. Saving those moments, embracing the process, and honoring your growth is where transformation truly happens.

If we do the work—if we trust, obey, and allow the Spirit to guide us—we are guaranteed to come out better people. Growth is not optional; it is built into the process when we align ourselves with God's truth and power.

Deeper Reflection

• Where do you feel held back, and what strongholds—thoughts, behaviors, or patterns—might be influencing those areas? Consider how long they've been present, how they've shaped your choices or relationships, and how leaning on God's Spirit can help you move toward freedom.

• Where have you already experienced growth or breakthroughs, and how can you apply those lessons now? Reflect on small, consistent ways to obey God's Word daily, and consider areas where releasing control to Him could bring clarity, movement, or new opportunities.

• Write a prayer of invitation. A prayer of invitation is just that—you are inviting God to be with you in this process. It doesn't matter how you write it, and there's no "right" way. What matters is that it comes from your heart. You are asking God to guide you, stay with you, and speak to you through the Holy Spirit as you navigate this journey. When you invite God in, you are opening yourself up to His instruction. You are saying, "I am ready to hear from You. I am open to Your leading." I am reminded of a close friend whose son passed away. A few years later, she told me about a moment of clarity God gave her. She had been holding everything tightly—so protective and so in control of the situation. God showed her that He couldn't bless the situation fully if she was holding on so tightly. She had to let go, to release control, and trust Him to lead. That same principle applies here: we can't receive God's guidance if we are trying to do it all ourselves. We have to release control and open our hearts. Simply write a prayer of invitation. Tell God, in your own words, that you invite Him into this process. It is to help you process, reflect, and begin this journey with Him at the center.

Tool for Your Journey

Prayer Prompt: "Lord, help me to rely on Your Spirit rather than my own understanding. Teach me to trust Your guidance, embrace the process, and walk in the freedom You've already provided. Amen."

Verses for Study

John 8:32 (AMP): *"And you will know the Truth [regarding salvation], and the Truth will set you free [from the penalty of sin]."*

Zechariah 4:6 (AMP): *"Then he said to me, 'This [continuous supply of oil] is the word of the Lord to Zerubbabel, saying, 'Not by might, nor by power, but by My Spirit [of Whom the oil is a symbol],' says the Lord of hosts.'"*

Day 5:
Gratitude

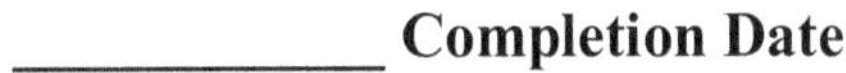

_________ Completion Date

Gratitude has the power to shift how we see the world. It's not about ignoring challenges or pretending life is perfect—it's about choosing to notice the blessings that are already present. Start small. Pay attention to everyday moments: the warmth of your morning coffee, the way your body moves as you stretch or walk, or even the simple completion of chores and responsibilities that might normally feel mundane. Each of these is an opportunity to pause and recognize God's goodness in your life.

Gratitude opens our hearts to God's presence and reminds us that He is actively at work, even in the small, ordinary moments. When we practice gratitude consistently, it reshapes our perspective, strengthens our faith, and equips us to respond with joy and contentment even in difficult circumstances.

Scripture Insight:

"Gratitude" appears in the Bible more than the word "thanks," 157 times. It's a recurring invitation to notice, acknowledge, and respond to God's gifts in every season of life.

Deeper Reflection

- Look up the definition of gratitude. Consider how it differs from simply saying "thank you" and how it relates to a heart fully aligned with God.
- Find Bible verses that mention gratitude. Reflect on

each verse and how it applies to your current season of life.

• Identify three things today—big or small—that you can actively be grateful for. Write them down and, if possible, reflect on how God's presence shows up through these blessings.

• How might intentionally noticing and acknowledging moments of gratitude change the way you approach your day, your challenges, or your relationships? Consider the perspective shift that gratitude can create, even in situations that feel routine or difficult.

Tools for Your Journey

Consider using this Daily Gratitude Tracker. In a notebook, write done the following headings, leaving a line for each one that you can write on:

Day: ____

Morning Moment: _________________________________

Body/Movement: __________________________________

Chores/Responsibilities: ___________________________

Other Blessings: ___________________________________

Verses for Study

1 Thessalonians 5:18 (AMP): *"In every situation [no matter what the circumstances] be thankful and continually give thanks to God; for this is the will of God for you in Christ Jesus."*

Colossians 3:15 (AMP): *"Let the peace of Christ [the inner calm of one who walks daily with Him] be the controlling factor in your hearts [deciding and settling questions that arise]. To this peace indeed you were called as members in one body [of believers]. And be thankful [to God always]."*

Day 6:
Trust the Process

_______________ **Completion Date**

Today, we focus on deepening our journey through two key practices: writing a prayer of affirmation and creating a struggle prayer. Each part is designed to strengthen your connection to God, reinforce self-discipline, and provide a foundation for growth.

Prayer of Affirmation

At first, affirmations can feel silly—telling yourself "I am this" or "I am that." But the truth is, you control what enters your mind. Your self-talk shapes your inner world, and no one else hears it. A prayer of affirmation is your way of claiming this journey for yourself and inviting God's presence into it daily. Write it down, place it where you'll see it every morning, or set a phone alarm to remind yourself.

A sample prayer might be: "God, I am free by Your power and Your Word. I believe You have given me the strength to break free from the bonds holding me back. I thank You that I am free through the sacrifice of Jesus. Empower me with Your wisdom and strength to be all You want me to be. In Jesus' name, Amen."

This practice renews your commitment daily, giving you a stable foundation to face challenges with confidence.

Even with affirmations, struggles are inevitable. You will face doubt, discouragement, or temptation to pull back. A struggle prayer acknowledges these moments honestly and invites God's guidance and strength. Think of it like having an emergency first-aid kit: you prepare for setbacks so you can respond thoughtfully rather than react impulsively.

Example: "Lord, I am struggling today. I feel discouraged and unsure, but I surrender this moment to You. Guide me, strengthen me, and help me persevere in the steps You've set before me. Amen."

By naming your struggles and praying through them, you exercise self-control and self-discipline while leaning on God's Spirit for support. Remember: struggles are normal. They are opportunities for growth, not signs of failure.

Deeper Reflection

- How can writing a daily prayer of affirmation change the way you start your day and influence your decisions?

- When you face struggles, how can you respond with intention rather than frustration? Consider how a prepared struggle prayer might support you in those moments.

Verses for Study

Philippians 4:13 (AMP): *"I can do all things [which He has called me to do] through Him who strengthens and empowers me [to fulfill His purpose—I am self-sufficient in Christ's sufficiency]; I am ready for anything and equal to anything through Him who infuses me with inner strength and confident peace."*

Isaiah 41:10 (AMP): *"Do not fear [anything], for I am with you; Do not be afraid, for I am your God. I will strengthen you, be assured I will help you; I will certainly take hold of you with My righteous right hand [a hand of justice, of power, of victory, of salvation]."*

Day 7:
The Power of Fellowship

_______________ **Completion Date**

Growth and transformation don't happen in isolation. Fellowship with others who share your goals, values, and faith strengthens your connection to God and provides encouragement along the way. Being part of a supportive community reminds us that we are not alone in our struggles or victories.

Even for those of us who are naturally private or introverted—like me—fellowship is essential. I am business-social, I love my family, and I deeply value my alone time. Yet, I've learned that even people who prefer solitude need community. Fellowship doesn't have to mean a super tight group of best friends who do everything together. In fact, that can feel overwhelming or uncomfortable.

Fellowship looks different for everyone. For some, it's a weekly small group or Bible study. For others, it's a consistent circle of friends you can check in with, share prayer requests, or celebrate wins. It could be a fitness class, a craft group, or volunteering in your church. It does not mean joining every group at church or overloading your schedule—fellowship does not need to be a monumental action, but rather meaningful connection. The key is that it provides encouragement, accountability, and shared energy—without pressure to conform to someone else's idea of connection.

Fellowship is more than casual connection; it creates accountability, reinforces faith, and multiplies motivation. Even small acts—offering a prayer, sharing an insight, or simply showing up—can have a profound impact. Your presence matters, and so does the encouragement you receive in return. Through fellowship, your journey becomes richer, lighter, and more deeply rooted in faith.

Reflection Prompts

- Who in your life reflects the kind of faith, focus, and encouragement you want to cultivate? How can you engage with them this week? Note: This person does not need to be part of your daily life, nor do you need to know them personally.

- What small ways can you participate in community to strengthen your connection with God and with others on a similar path?

Verses for Study

Hebrews 10:24-25 (AMP): *"And let us consider [thoughtfully] how we may encourage one another to love and to do good deeds, not forsaking our meeting together [as believers for worship and instruction], as is the habit of some, but encouraging one another; and all the more [faithfully] as you see the day [of Christ's return] approaching."*

Ecclesiastes 4:9-10 (AMP): *"Two are better than one because they have a more satisfying return for their labor; for if either of them falls, the one will lift up his companion. But woe to him who is alone when he falls and does not have another to lift him up."*

*Consider fellowshipping with me, Coach Cathleen and the rest of The Bodybuilding Potter community, called Team Emerge. You will find links and information at the end of this book.

Day 8:
Anchoring Your Journey

___________ Completion Date

Day 8 is about anchoring your foundation—think bedrock. Just as a skyscraper cannot stand on shifting sand, your health journey cannot stand without a strong, steady base. That base isn't just about physical habits—it's about mindset and spiritual grounding. When storms come, bedrock holds.

As a master potter, I see this same principle every time I sit at the wheel. Before anything beautiful is formed, the clay must be **centered**—anchored in the middle of the wheel. If it's even slightly off-center, the whole piece will wobble, warp, or collapse under pressure. This centering is the pottery version of laying bedrock—it's the non-negotiable starting point.

After shaping comes drying, trimming, and the first firing—transforming fragile clay into hardened ceramic. But it's still not done. Only after glazing and a final fire in the kiln does the vessel reach its full beauty and strength—ready to hold, to serve, and to be a testimony to the process it endured.

Your health journey is no different. You begin by anchoring yourself in truth. You *will* go through "ugly" stages where progress feels slow or invisible. But each step—each small habit, each moment of self-control, each focus of gratitude, and each surrender - becomes part of your foundation. Eventually, the foundation begins to take shape.

And here's a thought: "savor" and "Savior" are only one letter apart. To savor means to fully experience and appreciate each moment. When we savor our journey, we invite our

Savior into it—turning the process itself into a place of connection, trust, and transformation.

Deeper Reflection

- Reflect on one area of your health journey that feels "ugly" or still in progress, and write it down. Then, note why you will trust the process and commit to growth in that area.

- Look up the definitions of *savor* and *Savior* and create a short reflection, sentence, or poem connecting the two.

Verses for Study

Matthew 6:34 (AMP): *"So do not worry about tomorrow; for tomorrow will worry about itself. Each day has enough trouble of its own."*

Isaiah 64:8 (AMP): *"Yet, O Lord, You are our Father; We are the clay, and You our Potter, And we all are the work of Your hand."*

Day 9:
Building – Milk versus Meat: Self-Control

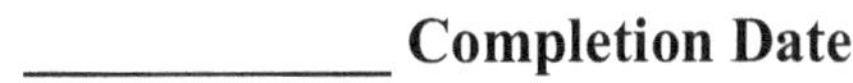

_____________ **Completion Date**

When you give a baby milk, it's exactly what they need at that stage—simple nourishment. But as the baby grows, gets teeth, and matures, his or her body needs something deeper—meat.

Babies don't jump from milk to meat—they move gradually, learning to take in more as they grow. A walk with Christ works the same way. When we first come to know God—whether as a child or an adult—we start with milk. The lighter lessons, like Noah's ark, the Christmas story, or simply learning that God loves us, are powerful truths, but they're just the beginning.

As we mature in our faith, God calls us to go deeper. Milk can only take us so far—we need the meat of Scripture, the more challenging lessons that stretch us, shape us, and grow us. This is also how we dig the foundation for a God-centered life. Each stage builds strength, laying the bedrock that will carry us through challenges, growth, and victories alike.

You are developing your spiritual teeth and through this work you've begun laying your foundation. Now it's time to dig into the deeper lesson of self-control.

Definition: Self-control is the ability to regulate your thoughts, emotions, and actions, choosing what honors God rather than what feels impulsive. Simply put, it means "stop." Stop before reacting, stop before giving in, and stop before making a choice that doesn't honor God or your body.

A Fruit of the Spirit: Self-control is not something you have to search for or earn—it is a fruit of the Spirit. You are born with it in Christ, and it only needs to be developed and practiced. The more you exercise it, the stronger it becomes.

Self-control is the cornerstone of progress. Every decision you make shapes your health, mind, and spirit. The Bible reminds us in Galatians 5:22-23 that self-control is a fruit of the Spirit—a power we can cultivate, not merely a limitation.

Examples of self-control in action:
- Stopping before snapping at a family member and choosing a gentle word instead.
- Stopping before eating something you know will harm your health and choosing a nourishing option.
- Stopping before scrolling through social media aimlessly and choosing prayer or Scripture reading.

With God at the center, learning to stop is not restrictive—it's freeing. It gives you space to respond intentionally and live with purpose.

Deeper Reflection

- Where in your life do you need to practice stopping before reacting, eating, or making a choice? Write one example.

- Choose one area of your health or faith where stopping will make the biggest difference. Write a practical step you will take this week to begin exercising self-control in that area.

Verse for Study

Hebrews 5:13–14 (AMP): *"For everyone who lives on milk is [doctrinally inexperienced and unskilled] in the word of righteousness, since he is a spiritual infant. But solid food is for the [spiritually] mature, whose senses are trained by practice to distinguish between what is morally good and what is evil."*

Day 10:
Building – Self-Discipline

__________ **Completion Date**

If self-control is about learning to stop, self-discipline is about learning to go. It is the action that follows your choice to honor God, your body, and your purpose. Whereas self-control helps you pause before making a wrong choice, self-discipline moves you forward to do what is right—even when it's hard, inconvenient, or uncomfortable.

Definition: Self-discipline is the ability to intentionally direct your actions toward a goal or standard, following through even when you don't feel like it. In its simplest form, it means "go."

Self-discipline builds on self-control. Once you stop impulsive behavior, self-discipline is what moves you to replace it with a healthy, God-honoring action. It turns intention into action, choice into habit, and small steps into lasting growth.

Even when your body is sore, your mind tempted, or motivation low, choosing discipline over indulgence is the key to long-term success.

Using self-discipline with the self-control Examples from Day 10:

- Reacting to a family member: Self-control stops the snap; self-discipline moves you to speak a gentle word or encourage them intentionally.

- Choosing what to eat: Self-control stops the unhealthy choice; self-discipline moves you to prepare or choose a nourishing meal.

- Using time wisely: Self-control stops the aimless

scrolling; self-discipline moves you to read Scripture, pray, or engage in something productive.

When practiced consistently, self-discipline strengthens your spiritual, emotional, and physical life. Like a muscle, it grows each time you choose to go where God calls you, even when it's difficult.

Deeper Reflection

- Think of one area in your health, relationships, or faith where you often stop but don't go. How can you apply self-discipline to move forward in that area?
- Identify a small, specific action you can take daily to exercise self-discipline, building strength and growth over time.

Verse for Study

Proverbs 25:28 (AMP): *"Like a city that is broken down and without walls [leaving it unprotected] Is a man who has no self-control over his spirit [and sets himself up for trouble]."*

Days 1 to 10:
Dig Deeper Day

_______________ **Completion Date**

Pause & Review

This is not a reset—it's a reminder of how far you've come and where God is still leading. Each day you've completed is not a checkmark of completion but another layer added to your lifelong healthy foundation in God.

On this day, pause and look back over all the work you've done so far. Notice the patterns God is weaving, the lessons that repeat, and the areas where your strength and faith are growing. Take time to adjust, change, and update your responses as you feel led—this is a journey of ongoing refinement.

Helpful Reflection Prompts

1. What have I learned about God through my journey so far?

2. How have I seen growth in my body, mind, and spirit from Day 1 until now?

3. What themes or lessons keep resurfacing, showing me where God is calling me to go deeper?

4. What practices or insights do I want to carry with me into the next stage of the journey?

Day 11:
Intro Fruits of the Spirit: Love

_______________ Completion Date

Now that you have a better understanding of self-control, it's time to step back and see the bigger picture. Self-control doesn't exist in isolation. These fruits are woven into the fabric of your spirit, not something you have to search for—they are already within you, ready to be nurtured and refined.

The Fruits of the Spirit are qualities that blossom in believers who are guided by the Holy Spirit. They shape your character, influence your choices, and reveal God's presence in your life. Here is the verse again (are you getting its importance) Galatians 5:22–23 lists them: love, joy, peace, patience, kindness, goodness, faithfulness, gentleness, and self-control.

Notice the order: love is first, and self-control is last, acting as bookends. Love supports the growth of all other fruits, while self-control ensures they remain upright and enduring—like a finely crafted bookshelf, each piece in perfect balance.

Love is the foundation, the heartbeat, and is the first listed.

Love is defined as intentional, selfless care for others, rooted in God's heart. It is the foundation of all spiritual growth, guiding every action, thought, and choice. Love is active, not passive—it sees beyond personal desire, seeks the good of others, and sustains every other fruit of the Spirit. It is patient, kind, forgiving, and steadfast, forming the soil from which all other virtues blossom.

Love Story

Imagine a master potter at the wheel. The clay is soft, waiting to be shaped. Love is the hands of the potter, gently guiding, molding, and forming the clay into something beautiful and strong. Every other emerges from the care and intention of these hands. Without love as the guiding touch, the clay remains shapeless, brittle, or cracked. Love is intentional, selfless, and deeply rooted. It calls you to shape your life and relationships with tenderness, to serve, to bless, and to act with purpose and care.

Deeper Reflection

Reflect on how love is showing up in your daily life.

Day 12:
Joy, Peace, and Patience

__________ **Completion Date**

The fruits of joy, peace, and patience cultivate a tranquil and radiant inner life, even amidst the chaos of the world.

Story / Reflection

Imagine sitting at the potter's wheel, the clay spinning steadily beneath your hands.

Joy is the vibrant details the potter adds to the clay, giving it life and brilliance even before it is fully formed. Peace is the steady rhythm of the wheel, allowing the clay to rotate without cracking, creating harmony in every turn. Patience is the careful touch, guiding the clay slowly, understanding it cannot be rushed without compromising its integrity.

Even when the wheel wobbles or the clay resists, these fruits keep your spirit steady, allowing the beauty of your life to emerge gracefully.

These fruits work together, helping you respond with grace when life tests your endurance. Even small moments of choosing joy, peace, or patience ripple outward, shaping your character and relationships.

Joy is **an inner delight and fullness of spirit** that persists regardless of circumstances. It is rooted in God's presence and promises, not fleeting feelings or temporary pleasures. Joy colors life with gratitude, celebration, and hope, even in moments of challenge. Like a vibrant glaze on pottery, joy brings warmth and brilliance to every aspect of your spiritual life.

Peace is **a deep, unshakable calm of the soul**, flowing from trust in God. It steadies your heart amid life's storms, quiets anxious thoughts, and restores clarity in the midst of chaos. Peace acts as the wheel that keeps the clay centered—steadying, aligning, and sustaining your spiritual formation.

Patience is **the gentle endurance that allows growth and transformation to unfold in God's timing**. It is the ability to wait without frustration, to respond with grace, and to persevere when progress feels slow. Patience is the tender touch of the potter, shaping the clay with care and precision, understanding that true beauty emerges over time.

Deeper Reflection

- Observe how joy is showing up in your life or is desired.

- Observe how peace is showing up in your life or is desired.

- Observe how patience is showing up in your life or is desired.

Day 13:
Kindness and Goodness

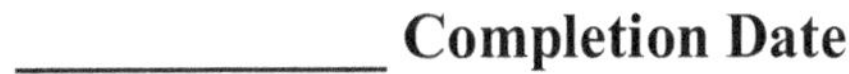

___________ Completion Date

Kindness and goodness shape your outward expressions and when exercised can create ripples of grace in the lives around you.

Story / Reflection

Picture a beautifully glazed clay mug sitting on a kitchen counter. The morning sunlight bounces off of its shiny surface. This is how the light will reflect off of someone who exercises kindness and goodness.

- Kindness is the warm glow. This glow can be felt by others in a soft yet profound way.
- Goodness is the clear integrity that shines through your actions.

When you practice kindness and goodness, you not only bless others but cultivate a spirit of generosity and peace within yourself. These fruits often require self-control to act rightly, especially when the natural impulse leans toward self-interest or inaction – both of which are part of human nature.

Deeper Reflection

- Small and large acts have rippling effects. Choose one act of kindness or goodness to do today. Let it flow naturally from the love that anchors you.
- Observe then detail how your small acts of care impact others and enrich your own spiritual walk.

Day 14:
Faithfulness and Gentleness

______________ **Completion Date**

Story / Reflection

Faithfulness and gentleness anchor your consistency and guide your attitude.

Faithfulness is the potter who shows up each day, tending to every step of the process—preparing and wedging the clay, shaping, drying, glazing, and firing—never abandoning the work until it is complete.

Gentleness is found in the potters' hands as they carefully sand the surface ensuring the vessel is ready for the next step in its journey – this requires care rather than force. Together, they reveal that true strength lies not in rushing or harshness, but in steady commitment and tender grace.

These fruits help you live a faith-filled life, even when circumstances are challenging or when others test your patience. They are cultivated through daily choices, guided by love and secured by self-control.

Deeper Reflection

• Identify one area where you can demonstrate faithfulness this week, honoring God and your commitments.

• Seek one opportunity to respond with gentleness, especially in a situation that tests you.

Day 15:
Fruits of the Spirit Review

_______________ **Completion Date**

With all of the fruits examined, let's work to integrate them into a vibrant, living practice.

Story / Reflection

Picture a bookshelf with each fruit being a book. Each of which is thickly-bound, vibrant and well used. The book collection includes: love, joy, peace, patience, kindness, goodness, faithfulness, gentleness, and self-control.

- The *Love* book is first in the collection. It is standing strong. It is the starting point for all of the other books to lean against.
- The *Joy* book is second in the collection. It is vibrant in color and finish offering light and resilience.
- The *Peace* book is third. It is soft in tone providing a calm presence.
- The *Patience* book is fourth. It is also soft in tone with many blank pages between the chapters.
- The *Kindness* book is fifth in the collection. It is finished in a glowing tone providing warmth to all who come near.
- The *Goodness* book is sixth in the collection. It has a clear book cover showing intention.
- The *Faithfulness* book is seventh in the collection. It is finished with visible dividers showing repetitiveness and returning.
- The *Gentleness* book is eight in the collection. It is

finished in a lavender quilt providing a soft touch.

- *Self-Control* book is in the ninth and last position. Keeping everything balanced and ensuring beauty and strength endure.

Deeper Reflection

Create a visual representation of the Fruits of the Spirit—poster board, notebook, or digital tools. Place love as the first book and self-control as the last. Arrange the other fruits in order. Work to focus on understanding and internalizing the fruits, not artistic perfection.

I would love to see your finished artwork. Please consider submitting to me at *cathleen@thebodybuildingpotter.com*.

Reflect and note what this Deeper Reflection taught you.

Day 16:
Savoring Growth

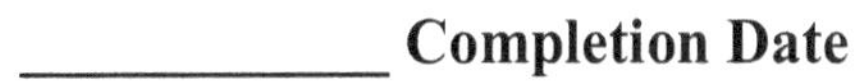 **Completion Date**

It is my hope that this day you will give yourself grace in the mess and take time to reflect on progress. Progress is rarely instant and instant progress does not have roots. Your body, mind, and spirit grow incrementally. The more we trust God and the more we see Him come through the easier is becomes to savor the process and keeps up engaged and resilient.

Deeper Reflection

- Identify 2 to 3 small changes you've made since starting this journey and identify how they have helped you dig deeper into your God-centered healthy lifestyle journey.

- How will you carry these practices into the coming week?

Day 17:
Choosing Discomfort

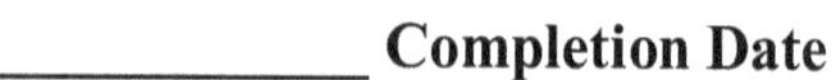

___________ Completion Date

Growth requires discomfort. Transformation doesn't happen in the comfort zone—it happens when we step into the spaces that stretch us, challenge us, and draw us to rely on God more fully.

Think about a seed planted in the soil. At first, it's buried in darkness, pressed down by dirt. If the seed could express feeling, it might experience discomfort or even a sense of being crushed. Yet, that very pressure is what allows it to break open, take root, and grow upward toward the light. Without discomfort, it would never become what it was created to be.

Our growth works the same way. When we cling only to what feels safe or easy, we remain unchanged. But when we step into discomfort—whether it's a new discipline, a shift in habit, or a spiritual challenge—we open ourselves to God's transforming work.

Deeper Reflection

- Where in your life do you tend to avoid discomfort? (You're eating habits, workout consistency, or prayer life?)
- Ask: What area is God inviting you to step into—even if it feels uncomfortable—so that you can grow?
- Write down one place you will intentionally choose discomfort this week, trusting that God will meet you there.

Verse for Study

2 Corinthians 12:9-10 (AMP): *"But He has said to me,*

'My grace is sufficient for you [My lovingkindness and My mercy are more than enough—always available—regardless of the situation]; for [My] power is being perfected [and is completed and shows itself most effectively] in [your] weakness.' Therefore, I will all the more gladly boast in my weaknesses, so that the power of Christ [may completely enfold me and] may dwell in me.

"So I am well pleased with weaknesses, with insults, with distresses, with persecutions, and with difficulties, for the sake of Christ; for when I am weak [in human strength], then I am strong [truly able, truly powerful, truly drawing from God's strength]."

Day 18:

Progress, Not Perfection

_________ **Completion Date**

Transformation is progress, not perfection. Growth isn't about getting everything right all the time—it's about taking intentional steps, leaning on God's grace, and steadily moving forward.

Think about building a foundation for a home. You don't start with the walls or the roof; you begin with small, careful steps, preparing—laying bricks, leveling, and reinforcing the structure. Each brick might not be perfect, but over time, those imperfect bricks form something strong and lasting.

Our lives work the same way. In health, fitness, and faith, there will be days when you fall short or make mistakes. That doesn't mean failure—it's part of the process. Each intentional choice, each disciplined action, adds up over time. The key is consistency, not perfection.

Deeper Reflection

- Where in your life are you expecting perfection instead of progress? (Workouts, nutrition, prayer life, or spiritual growth?)

- Identify one area where you can focus on small, consistent steps this week.

- Write down one action you will take each day, remembering that God honors effort and faithfulness more than flawless execution.

Verse for Study

Galatians 6:9 (AMP): *"Let us not grow weary or become discouraged in doing good, for at the proper time we will reap, if we do not give in."*

Day 19:
The Power of Small Habits

________________ **Completion Date**

Small habits matter. The little choices we make every day build the foundation for lasting change in our health, fitness, and spiritual life.

Think about putting away your dishes or tidying your workspace each day. It may seem insignificant in the moment, but over time, these small acts create order, discipline, and momentum. Like a single drop of water creating ripples, small habits compound into larger transformation.

In the same way, consistently choosing prayer, movement, or nutritious meals—even when it feels minor or tedious—strengthens your ability to tackle bigger challenges. These "tiny victories" become the stepping stones for long-term growth.

Deeper Reflection

- Identify one small habit this week you can commit to consistently—something that may feel minor but will have a meaningful impact over time.
- How can you make that habit part of your daily routine?
- Write down your plan and focus on doing it consistently, trusting God to multiply your efforts into bigger change.

Day 20:
Faithfulness in the Little Things

_____________ **Completion Date**

Similarly to Day 19, faithfulness in small things prepares you for greater responsibilities. Being consistent and disciplined in the small tasks of life builds character, trust, and readiness for bigger challenges.

Luke 16:10–13 (AMP) says: *"He who is faithful in a very little thing is also faithful in much; and he who is dishonest in a very little thing is also dishonest in much. Therefore if you have not been faithful in the use of earthly wealth, who will entrust the true riches to you? And if you have not been faithful in the use of that [earthly wealth] which belongs to another [whether God or man, and of which you are a trustee], who will give you that which is your own? No servant can serve two masters; for either he will hate the one and love the other, or he will stand devotedly by the one and despise the other. You cannot serve God and mammon [that is, your earthly possessions or anything else you trust in and rely on instead of God]."*

Your consistency in daily acts of faith and discipline reflects your character. Over time, these small choices accumulate and prepare you to handle larger opportunities and responsibilities.

Deeper Reflection
- Look at the small, everyday tasks in your life. Where

can you be more faithful and consistent?

- Choose one "small thing" this week to focus on and commit to doing it diligently.
- Reflect on how practicing faithfulness in little things strengthens your discipline and prepares you for bigger blessings from God.

Days 1 to 20:
Dig Deeper Day

______________ Completion Date

Pause & Review

This is not a reset—it's a reminder of how far you've come and where God is still leading. Each day you've completed is not a checkmark of completion but another layer added to your lifelong healthy foundation in God.

On this day, pause and look back over all the work you've done so far. Notice the patterns God is weaving, the lessons that repeat, and the areas where your strength and faith are growing. Take time to adjust, change, and update your responses as you feel led—this is a journey of ongoing refinement.

Helpful Reflection Prompts

1. What have I learned about God through my journey so far?

2. How have I seen growth in my body, mind, and spirit from Day 1 until now?

3. What themes or lessons keep resurfacing, showing me where God is calling me to go deeper?

4. What practices or insights do I want to carry with me into the next stage of the journey?

Day 21:
Acting in Truth, Not Just Feelings

______________ **Completion Date**

Feelings are real, but they don't define the truth. Our emotions can fluctuate, but God's Word and His promises remain constant. Learning to act in alignment with truth, not just how we feel, is essential for growth and discipline.

Imagine waking up feeling unmotivated, discouraged, or frustrated. You might feel like skipping a workout, ignoring your prayer time, or abandoning a goal. These feelings are valid—they're part of being human—but they are not the ultimate authority.

Acting in discipline, guided by faith and truth, allows us to rise above temporary emotions. When we choose to move forward despite our feelings, we grow stronger spiritually, mentally, and physically.

Deeper Reflection

• Think about an area where your feelings often dictate your actions—maybe skipping a workout, avoiding prayer, or indulging in a habit you want to change.

• Ask: What is the truth in this situation according to God's Word and my long-term goals?

• Commit to acting in alignment with that truth this week, even if your feelings resist.

Verse for Study

Proverbs 3:5 (AMP): *"Trust in and rely confidently on the Lord with all your heart and do not rely on your own insight or understanding."*

Day 22:
Self-Discipline as a Pathway to Freedom

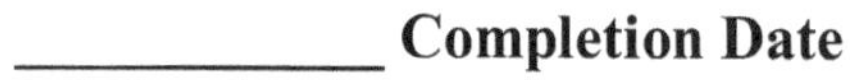

__________ **Completion Date**

Self-control and self-discipline are not limitations—they are pathways to freedom. Choosing to act intentionally, rather than react impulsively, allows you to live with purpose and experience true liberty in your health, habits, and faith.

Think about the simple exercise of "put it away, don't put it down." At first, it seems trivial or even restrictive. But practicing this discipline in small ways trains your mind and heart to make intentional choices. Over time, this builds the strength to make larger decisions wisely—choosing nutritious meals, consistent workouts, or daily prayer even when it feels inconvenient.

The paradox is clear: the more we practice self-control and self-discipline, the more freedom we gain. We are no longer slaves to impulses, emotions, or habits; instead, we live intentionally in alignment with God's plan.

Deeper Reflection

- Identify one area in your life where exercising self-control feels difficult.
- Commit to applying discipline in that area this week. You are highly encouraged to incorporate PIA-DPID (Put it away, don't put it down) in to your daily acts of discipline.
- Notice how taking intentional action, even in small ways, creates a sense of freedom and empowerment. Reflect

on how God uses self-discipline to guide you toward the life He desires for you.

Verse for Study

Proverbs 25:28 (AMP): *"Like a city that is broken down and without walls [leaving it unprotected] Is a man who has no self-control over his spirit [and sets himself up for trouble]."*

Day 23:

Purpose-Driven Motivation

__________ **Completion Date**

Motivation and willpower are often treated as dependable forces, yet they are inconsistent and unreliable. Many people wait to feel motivated before taking action, only to find that those feelings fade when discomfort appears. If progress depends on how we feel in the moment, growth becomes fragile and inconsistent.

Motivation is most lasting when it comes from purpose, not fleeting feelings. Your "why"—your faith, goals, and God-given vision—drives consistent action, even on days when you don't feel like it.

Imagine waking up early for an important day, even though it's cold, you're tired, and all you want is coffee in bed. Your feelings might beg you to stay home, but your purpose—your desire to honor God with your health, reach your goals, or inspire others—keeps you moving.

Relying solely on feelings makes progress inconsistent. Purpose gives you a reason to act beyond temporary emotions. Each step you take toward your "why," even when uncomfortable, compounds into growth, discipline, and transformation.

Deeper Reflection

- Reflect on one area where your feelings often dictate your actions.

- What is your deeper purpose in this area? Write down your "why."

- Plan one intentional action this week to honor that

purpose, even if it doesn't feel easy.

Verse for Study

Proverbs 16:3 (AMP): *"Commit your works to the Lord [submit and trust them to Him], And your plans will succeed [if you respond to His will and guidance]."*

Day 24:
Strengthening Your Foundation

______________ **Completion Date**

The foundation of any health or fitness journey is not just what you eat or how you move—it's your heart, your mindset, and your faith. When I first started this journey, I thought that working out harder or eating "perfectly" would bring results. But without the core principles—self-control, self-discipline, gratitude, faith, and focus—I struggled to sustain anything.

It wasn't until I fully surrendered and committed to these foundational elements that my workouts became consistent, my nutrition mindful, and my spirit centered.

Deeper Reflection

- Examine your foundation. Where are you strong, and where might you need reinforcement?

- Are you practicing self-control with your choices, staying disciplined even when it's hard, and keeping a heart of gratitude?

- Are your faith and focus guiding your actions? Write down one area you want to strengthen this week and ask God to guide you.

Verse for Study

Matthew 7:24 (AMP): *"So everyone who hears these words of Mine and acts on them, will be like a wise man [a farsighted, practical, and sensible man] who built his house on the rock."*

Day 25:
Moving at Your Own Pace

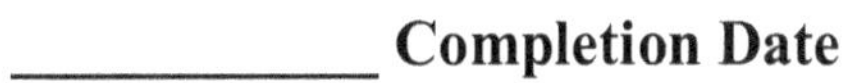

__________ Completion Date

It can be tempting to rush into a "perfect" fitness or nutrition plan, especially with all the worldly noise about what you "should" do. When I first started, I wanted to try every method, every supplement, and every "quick fix." But rushing before you are truly ready for physical transformation will only lead to frustration.

God reminds us that this journey is about you—not your friends, not your family, not what anyone else is doing. He gave you this body, this life, and this time to care for yourself as He designed. When your heart, mind, and faith are aligned, the steps you take will stick.

Deeper Reflection

- Ask yourself: Am I truly ready to take the next step in my health and fitness journey, or am I rushing to keep up with others?
- Pause and listen to your body and spirit.
- Identify one area where you feel ready to take action and commit it to God.

Verse for Study

Psalm 27:14 (AMP): *"Wait for and confidently expect the Lord; Be strong and let your heart take courage; Yes, wait for and confidently expect the Lord."*

Day 26:
Filtering the Noise

_______________ **Completion Date**

There is so much noise about health, fitness, and nutrition—from miracle supplements to trending diets. It can feel overwhelming and discouraging. Quick fixes don't last. Sustainability comes from building a solid foundation rooted in self-control, self-discipline, gratitude, faith, and focus. God has equipped us with everything we need; the rest is distractions. Distractions are designed to pull you away from the goals at hand. Pay attention!

Deeper Reflection

- Identify one "noise" in the health and fitness world that tempts you.
- Write down why it isn't aligned with God's plan for your body and life.
- Replace that thought with a principle rooted in faith, self-discipline, or gratitude. Filtering the noise creates mental and spiritual space to pursue true goals.

Verse for Study

Romans 12:2 (AMP): *"And do not be conformed to this world [any longer with its superficial values and customs], but be transformed and progressively changed [as you mature spiritually] by the renewing of your mind [focusing on godly values and ethical attitudes], so that you may prove [for yourselves] what the will of God is, that which is good and acceptable and perfect [in His plan and purpose for you]."*

Day 27:
Purpose-Driven Fitness and Nutrition

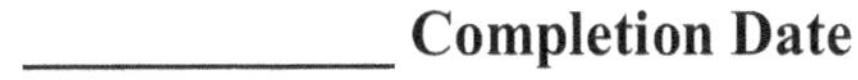 **Completion Date**

Everything—even our health and fitness—is tied to a bigger purpose. We aren't promised tomorrow, and every choice matters. Every stretch, meal, and workout can be an act of worship, a way to honor God by stewarding the gift He's given us. It's not about perfection—it's about purpose.

Deeper Reflection

- Reflect on why you want to be healthy and fit beyond appearance.
- How can your choices reflect gratitude, faith, and obedience to God?
- Write down your purpose for learning to move your body and fueling it well. Let this purpose guide your decisions this week.

Verse for Study

1 Corinthians 10:31 (AMP): *"So then, whether you eat or drink or whatever you do, do all to the glory of [our great] God."*

Day 28:
Movement as Medicine

_____________ **Completion Date**

I started my fitness journey with yoga, spending just 10 minutes a day focusing on my core and spinal muscles. Simple movements, such as the cobra pose, strengthened my back and supported my body in ways I didn't realize I needed. These movements taught me patience, mindfulness, and breathing control—skills that translated into mental and spiritual growth as well.

It is important to pause here. For many Christians, the word _yoga_ raises concern—and rightly so, as yoga as a spiritual practice has roots outside of Christianity. What I am referring to, however, is not a spiritual ritual, but the physical movement aspect only. Stretching, strengthening, and breathing exercises are simply ways of caring for the body God gave us. Just as lifting weights or taking a walk can honor God, so can mindful stretching when done with the intention of glorifying Him rather than engaging another belief system.

Even when life became busy, I made space for this practice each morning, pairing it with prayerful meditation and reflection. These small, consistent steps became a foundation for larger fitness goals.

Deeper Reflection

- Prioritize gentle movement that strengthens and centers you today whether it's yoga, stretching, or a short walk, notice how it makes your body feel and how it connects you to God.

- Consistency, even in small amounts, creates a foundation for growth—physically and spiritually.

Verse for Study

1 Corinthians 6:19 (AMP): *"Do you not know that your body is a temple of the Holy Spirit who is within you, whom you have [received as a gift] from God, and that you are not your own [property]?"*

Day 29:
Entering the "Gym" with Confidence

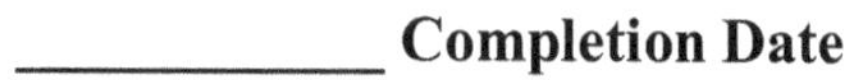

_________________ **Completion Date**

After building a base with yoga, I joined the gym. At first, I was nervous and intimidated, unsure of how to use the equipment or where to start. It had been many years since I was in a public gym. I took time to explore, learn each machine, and gradually gain confidence. I didn't push myself to extremes or rush progress; instead, I focused on understanding my body, enjoying movement, and giving myself grace. Over time, what once felt overwhelming became familiar, empowering, and even enjoyable.

Deeper Reflection

- Approach new environments with curiosity rather than fear.

- Explore your current or potential fitness space, learn the tools available, and celebrate small victories. I personally work out at home.

- Confidence grows through consistent exposure and grace, not perfection. Trust that God equips you to take the first step, and each step builds your foundation.

Verse for Study

Philippians 4:13 (AMP): *"I can do all things [which He has called me to do] through Him who strengthens and empowers me [to fulfill His purpose—I am self-sufficient in*

Christ's sufficiency]; I am ready for anything and equal to anything through Him who infuses me with inner strength and confident peace."

Day 30:
Mindful Eating
and Personalized Nutrition

__________ **Completion Date**

When I began focusing on nutrition, I started by simply becoming mindful of what I ate rather than following extreme plans. Later, I joined a food point–tracking program to gain a deeper understanding of portion sizes and food choices. While my goal was to lose fat, I also wanted to be fit and strong. I had a deep desire to understand how God specifically designed me—how He created me as His unique artwork with visible muscles and more.

To build muscle while losing fat, I learned more about both macro- and micronutrition. I learned how to eat in a macro-based way, focusing on balancing protein, carbohydrates, and fats to support my body and my goals.

Over time, I realized that nutrition is deeply personal—what works for me may not work for someone else. The key was building a foundation first, understanding my hunger cues, and adjusting as needed, always giving myself grace when things didn't go perfectly.

Deeper Reflection

- Consider your eating habits and how they support your goals.
- Focus on mindful choices, balance, and consistency rather than following a "one-size-fits-all" plan.
- Honor your body by listening, learning, and adjusting. Progress matters more than perfection.

Days 1 to 30:

Dig Deeper Day

__________ Completion Date

Pause & Review

This is not a reset—it's a reminder of how far you've come and where God is still leading. Each day you've completed is not a checkmark of completion but another layer added to your lifelong healthy foundation in God.

On this day, pause and look back over all the work you've done so far. Notice the patterns God is weaving, the lessons that repeat, and the areas where your strength and faith are growing. Take time to adjust, change, and update your responses as you feel led—this is a journey of ongoing refinement.

Helpful Reflection Prompts

1. What have I learned about God through my journey so far?

2. How have I seen growth in my body, mind, and spirit from Day 1 until now?

3. What themes or lessons keep resurfacing, showing me where God is calling me to go deeper?

4. What practices or insights do I want to carry with me into the next stage of the journey?

Day 31:
Building a Sustainable Routine

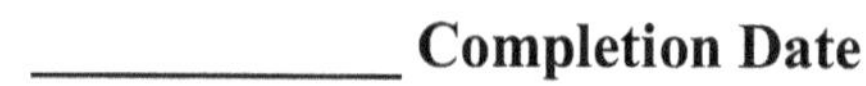 **Completion Date**

As I progressed in my journey, I realized that fitness and nutrition work best when they are sustainable and personalized. The BEST routine is always one you can stick with. I combined daily yoga for strength and flexibility, regular gym sessions for resistance training, and mindful nutrition practices. I learned that trying to do everything perfectly from the start only leads to burnout. Over time, by staying consistent and listening to my body, I saw lasting changes—not just in my physique but in my energy, confidence, and mental health.

Deeper Reflection

• Reflect on your own routine or what you desire in a routine: what small, consistent steps can you take to integrate movement and mindful eating into your life?

• Focus on sustainability rather than perfection.

• God gives us the discipline, focus, and perseverance to honor our bodies daily. Faithful, steady steps forward lead to lasting change.

Verse for Study

Galatians 6:9 (AMP): *"Let us not grow weary or become discouraged in doing good, for at the proper time we will reap, if we do not give in."*

Day 32:
Visualizing Your Healthy Self

__________ **Completion Date**

One of the most powerful exercises on this journey is closing your eyes and truly seeing your healthiest, strongest version. Picture yourself in the gym, moving with confidence, feeling energized and capable. Notice how your clothes fit, the strength in your movements, and the pride in your posture. This isn't about comparing yourself to anyone else—it's about seeing the attainable version of YOU and using that vision to guide your daily choices.

Deeper Reflection

- Close your eyes and imagine your healthiest self. What do you look like?
- How do you feel when you move?
- What small habits can you build today to move closer to this version of you? Visualizing your best self honors God and gives clarity to your goals.

Verse for Study

Jeremiah 29:11 (AMP): *"For I know the plans and thoughts that I have for you,' says the Lord, 'plans for peace and well-being and not for disaster, to give you a future and a hope."*

Day 33:
Creating Your Own Fitness Routine

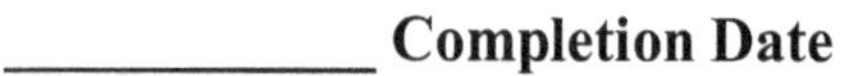 **Completion Date**

There's no one-size-fits-all approach to fitness. I started with yoga, just 10 minutes a day, focusing on strengthening my spine and core. When I was sick for 19 years, I had severe back pain. The last time I threw my back out I walked with a cane for two weeks. That small, consistent 10-minute effort became the foundation for everything else. Later, I joined a gym, taking time to learn each machine, exploring movements, and giving myself grace to grow into the routine. The key wasn't speed or intensity—it was consistency, curiosity, and honoring my body's limits while challenging it gently.

Deeper Reflection

- Your fitness routine should fit your life, goals, and abilities.
- Start small, focus on consistency, obedience in routine, and explore what works for you.
- Every movement is a way to honor God by caring for the body He gave you. Progress matters more than perfection.

Verse for Study

Hebrews 12:1 (AMP): *"Therefore, since we are surrounded by so great a cloud of witnesses [who by faith have testified to the truth of God's absolute faithfulness], stripping off every unnecessary weight and the sin which so easily and cleverly entangles us, let us run with endurance and active persistence the race that is set before us."*

Day 34:

Visualizing Your Healthy Self (Revisited)

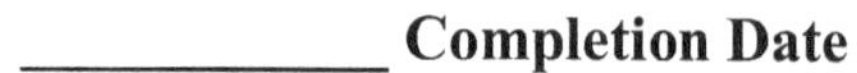 **Completion Date**

When I began my fitness journey, I realized it wasn't just about movement or nutrition—it was about clarity. I closed my eyes and pictured the healthiest version of myself: how she moved, how her clothes fit, how she felt in her body, and the confidence she carried. This visualization became a compass, guiding daily choices in fitness, nutrition, and self-care. It also needed to be realistic—reflecting my unique body, lifestyle, and goals, not a comparison to anyone else.

Deeper Reflection

- Visualizing your healthiest self gives you a concrete picture to work toward.
- What do you look like?
- What choices support your health and purpose? This clarity makes your journey intentional, rooted in gratitude, faith, focus, and self-discipline.

Verse for Study

Colossians 3:2 (AMP): *"Set your mind and keep focused habitually on the things above [the heavenly things], not on things that are on the earth [which have only temporal value]."*

Day 35:
Creating Obedience in a Sustainable Fitness Routine

______________ **Completion Date**

Obedience with consistency matters more than intensity. I started with small, sustainable actions: 10 minutes of yoga each morning for 6 weeks at 5 days a week. Only when I developed consistency in this routine did I add in going to the gym. I learned how to use gym equipment properly, and gradually adding strength training. Over time, these small, consistent steps built strength, confidence, and endurance. I learned to give myself grace—some days looked different than others, but showing up mattered most. I learned to give myself grace in the ebbs and flows of life.

Deeper Reflection

- What realistic steps can you take daily or weekly to honor your body and goals?
- Focus on consistency over intensity, learn your body, and give yourself grace.
- Sustainable routines strengthen your body, build confidence, and align with God-centered self-discipline, gratitude, and focus.
- How can you build obedience with your routine?

Day 36:
Mindful Nutrition and Personal Awareness

_______________ **Completion Date**

Mindful nutrition is about awareness, not perfection. What works well for someone else may not work for you—and that is okay. I began by paying attention to my choices rather than chasing food trends or extreme plans. Tracking portions, and later learning to understand macros, allowed me to fuel my body with intention rather than restriction.

Eating intentionally to fuel my body became a practical way to renew my mind, replacing emotionally driven choices with purposeful, God-honoring ones. Over time, I learned to listen to my body, recognize its unique needs, and make adjustments without judgment.

Tracking food is not a punishment—it is a tool. It is not about control or restriction, but about awareness and stewardship. Used with the right heart, tracking helped remove guesswork and guilt, replacing them with understanding and informed choice. It offered structure without shame and clarity without condemnation.

For me, learning about macronutrients became another helpful layer of understanding—not a rule to follow, but a framework to learn from. Understanding how protein, carbohydrates, and fats work together helped me support strength, energy, and overall health. This approach provided guidance without rigidity and allowed flexibility as I continued listening to my body and honoring how God designed me.

Deeper Reflection

- What does your body need today? How can you honor it with choices that fuel and strengthen you?

- Avoid the noise of trends and quick fixes—focus on what God has already provided: your amazing body and the wisdom to care for it.

- Developing this awareness builds self-control, gratitude, and confidence in your journey.

- How do you feel God is calling you to fuel your body in this season? What resources do you already have—or can seek out—to support that calling?

Day 37:
Visualizing Your Healthy Self (Revisited Again)

___________ **Completion Date**

One of the most powerful tools in my journey has been picturing my healthiest, strongest, most confident self. I remember sitting quietly and imagining what she looked like, how she moved, and how she felt in her own skin—not a celebrity, not someone else's ideal, but me at my best. This mental image guided my workouts, nutrition, and mindset. It kept me motivated, gave clarity to my choices, and reminded me that every small effort brought me closer to that version of myself.

Deeper Reflection

- Take time today to once again visualize your healthiest self.

- This isn't about perfection—it's about defining a goal, revisiting it often and making it attainable and meaningful to you.

- Let this vision guide your choices, remembering that faith, focus, self-discipline, and gratitude support every step toward becoming "you."

Day 38:
Making Time for Your Health

_____________ **Completion Date**

I used to think I didn't have time for the gym or consistent movement. Then I realized it wasn't about having time—it was about making time for what truly matters. Mornings became my dedicated hours for cardio or strength work, even if it meant waking before sunrise. I structured my day so that my health was a non-negotiable, essential part of life. The difference wasn't in having more hours; it was in prioritizing what mattered most.

Caring for your health is not selfish; it is an act of stewardship that positions you to show up more fully, serve more faithfully, and live with greater strength and clarity in every area of life.

Deeper Reflection

- Look at your schedule and identify where you can intentionally carve out time for your health.
- Even 10 minutes a day counts if done consistently.
- Decide what's essential for your physical and mental well-being, and commit to showing up for yourself. Remember: you are worth the time, and God gave you this body to care for and move with purpose.

Day 39:
Taking Action on Your Vision

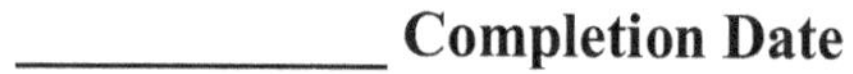

______________ **Completion Date**

Having a clear vision of your healthiest self is powerful—but it's only part of the journey. When I knew what I wanted to achieve, I realized I had to take consistent, small actions daily. Intentional prayer time, stretching in the morning, mindful meals, and learning the gym equipment became part of my routine. Some days were easier than others, but each step—no matter how small—brought me closer to my goal. Even when I was away from home, I adjusted and did what I could, trusting that consistency, not perfection, matters most.

Deeper Reflection

- Take one action today that aligns with your healthiest self.
- It doesn't have to be huge—just something that can be built into a consistent behavior.
- Reflect on how even small, faithful steps move you closer to your vision and honor the body God has given you.

Verse for Study

Colossians 3:23 (AMP): *"Whatever you do [whatever your task may be], work from the soul [that is, put in your very best effort], as [something done] for the Lord and not for men."*

Day 40:
Grace and Patience in Your Progress

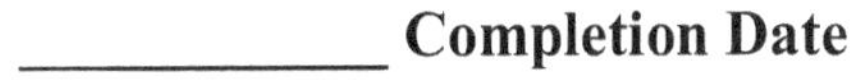
Completion Date

Sometimes we measure ourselves by other people's timelines or standards, but our journey is **uniquely ours**. I remember early in my training, comparing myself to others at the gym—it was overwhelming. Over time, I learned to give myself grace. Some days my workouts were shorter, my meals less perfect, but I stayed consistent. That grace allowed me to grow without discouragement, keeping faith that God's timing and my readiness matter more than perfection. I developed the confidence that I was being slowly refined by His teachings.

Deeper Reflection
- Reflect on where you might be too hard on yourself.
- Choose to extend grace to your efforts today.
- Celebrate the small wins, consistency, and faithfulness you are showing in caring for your body and walking with God. Progress isn't about perfection—it's about persistent steps forward.

Verse for Study
James 1:4 (AMP): *"And let endurance have its perfect result and do a thorough work, so that you may be perfect and completely developed [in your faith], lacking in nothing."*

Days 1 to 40:
Dig Deeper Day

____________ **Completion Date**

Pause & Review

This is not a reset—it's a reminder of how far you've come and where God is still leading. Each day you've completed is not a checkmark of completion but another layer added to your lifelong healthy foundation in God.

On this day, pause and look back over all the work you've done so far. Notice the patterns God is weaving, the lessons that repeat, and the areas where your strength and faith are growing. Take time to adjust, change, and update your responses as you feel led—this is a journey of ongoing refinement.

Helpful Reflection Prompts

1. What have I learned about God through my journey so far?

2. How have I seen growth in my body, mind, and spirit from Day 1 until now?

3. What themes or lessons keep resurfacing, showing me where God is calling me to go deeper?

4. What practices or insights do I want to carry with me into the next stage of the journey?

Day 41:
Identify the Noise and Stay Centered

_____________ **Completion Date**

There's an endless amount of health and fitness advice—quick fixes, supplements, trends—but most of it isn't sustainable. When I first started learning about nutrition, it was easy to get distracted by every new product or plan. Over time, I realized the key was identifying the noise and staying centered on the foundation: self-control, faith, gratitude, and focus. Filtering out distractions allowed me to make choices aligned with God's purpose for my body. This recognition changed my entire thought pattern.

Deeper Reflection

- Notice the "noise" around you—ads, trends, social media hype.
- Write down one thing that tempts you to stray from your healthy path.
- Ask: Is this truly honoring God and my goals? Refocus on what matters: your foundation.

Day 42:

Grace in Your Health and Fitness Journey

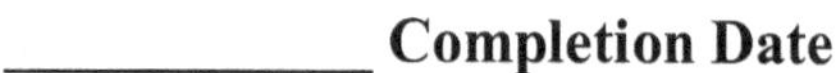 **Completion Date**

Even with a clear plan, life isn't always perfect. I remember being away from my usual routine, yet still committed to workouts and nutrition. Some days were harder than others, but I learned to give myself grace. I couldn't expect perfection every day, but I could keep showing up and doing my best. This mindset allowed me to grow stronger physically and spiritually, without guilt or frustration.

Life does not happen in a vacuum. Unexpected schedules, responsibilities, and disruptions will always exist. What I learned was to focus on what I *could* control rather than becoming discouraged by what I could not. I could choose my attitude, my effort, and my willingness to show up in whatever capacity the day allowed. By releasing the need to control everything and instead stewarding the choices within my reach, I found freedom, consistency, and peace in the process.

Deeper Reflection

- Reflect on areas where you may be too hard on yourself—movement, nutrition, or spiritual practices.
- Recognize that God's grace covers imperfections.
- Ask Him to help you embrace progress over perfection and celebrate every small step toward your goals.

Day 43:
Mental Toughness – Definition & Importance

______________ **Completion Date**

Mental toughness is the ability to handle stress, pressure, and challenges effectively. Jonah faced disappointment and stubbornness, while Job endured hopelessness, loss, and anguish. Their stories show that mental strength doesn't remove difficulty—it allows perseverance in the face of it. James reminds us, in James 1:12 (AMP): *"Blessed [happy, spiritually prosperous, favored by God] is the man who is steadfast under trial and perseveres when tempted; for when he has passed the test and been approved, he will receive the [victor's] crown of life which the Lord has promised to those who love Him."*

Deeper Reflection

1. How have you noticed your mental toughness being tested?

2. Which areas of your life feel the most mentally challenging?

3. How can understanding mental toughness help you approach challenges differently?

Assignment

- Look up the definition of mental toughness and write it down.

Day 44:
Mental Toughness in Daily Life & Mundanity

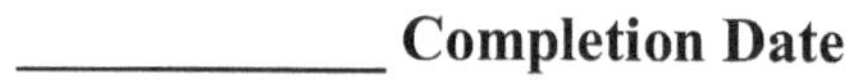

_____________ **Completion Date**

Mental toughness isn't just for crises—it's for everyday tasks. Even mundane routines like laundry, cooking, or workouts require strength and discipline. Naomi experienced grief, and Job endured daily suffering, yet both persisted. Their quiet perseverance shows that consistency in small actions prepares us for bigger challenges. As we have seen, 1 Corinthians 10:31 (AMP) reminds us, *"So then, whether you eat or drink or whatever you do, do all to the glory of [our great] God"* and Colossians 3:23 (AMP) adds, *"Whatever you do [whatever your task may be], work from the soul [that is, put in your very best effort], as [something done] for the Lord and not for men."*

Deeper Reflection

1.   Which mundane tasks challenge your consistency?

2.   How can you apply mental toughness to these daily routines?

3.   What small actions today can reinforce your discipline and resilience?

Assignment

•   Identify three daily routines that require mental toughness.

•   Track your consistency with these routines for a week.

Day 45:
Biblical Examples of Mental Strength

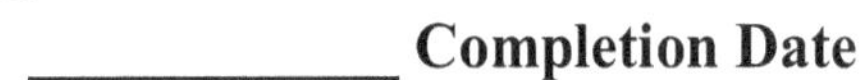

__________ Completion Date

The Bible is full of examples of resilience and persever-ance. Jonah's stubbornness taught him the importance of obedience, Job endured unimaginable loss but remained faithful, and Naomi's grief shows that life's struggles can weigh heavily but restoration is possible. Romans 5:3-4 (AMP) reminds us, *"And not only this, but with joy let us exult in our sufferings and rejoice in our hardships, knowing that hardship (distress, pressure, trouble) produces patient endurance; and endurance, proven character (spiritual maturity); and proven character, hope and confident assurance [of eternal salvation]"* and Psalm 34:19 (AMP) reassures us, *"Many hardships and perplexing circumstances confront the righteous, But the Lord rescues him from them all."*

Deeper Reflection

1. Research Jonah, Job, and Naomi and determine which Biblical story resonates most with your current challenges?

2. How did these figures demonstrate resilience in trials?

3. What lessons can you apply to your own mental toughness journey?

Day 46:

Spiritual Tools for Mental Strength (Part 1)

_____________ **Completion Date**

Mental toughness grows when paired with spiritual practices. Prayer, Scripture, and gratitude aren't just spiritual habits—they are mental tools. Job's faith and reflection show how connecting to God sustains resilience. Philippians 4:6-7 (AMP) encourages, *"Do not be anxious or worried about anything, but in everything [every circumstance and situation] by prayer and petition with thanksgiving, continue to make your [specific] requests known to God. And the peace of God [that peace which reassures the heart, that peace] which transcends all understanding, stands guard over your hearts and your minds in Christ Jesus."* 1 Thessalonians 5:16-18 (AMP) teaches, *"Rejoice always and delight in your faith; be unceasing and persistent in prayer; in every situation [no matter what the circumstances] be thankful and continually give thanks to God; for this is the will of God for you in Christ Jesus."*

Deeper Reflection

1. How can prayer help you maintain focus and strength during challenges?

2. Which scriptures have helped you persevere in the past?

3. How can practicing gratitude shift your perspective on daily struggles?

Assignment

- Spend 10–15 minutes in prayer today, focusing on mental strength.
- Write down three things you are grateful for and reflect on how they support your resilience.

Day 47:

Spiritual Tools for Mental Strength (Part 2)

_____________ **Completion Date**

Community, trust, and self-care reinforce mental toughness. As we have seen Ecclesiastes 4:9-10 (AMP) reminds us, *"Two are better than one because they have a more satisfying return for their labor; for if either of them falls, the one will lift up his companion. But woe to him who is alone when he falls and does not have another to lift him up."* Seeking support, trusting God's plan during highs and lows, and practicing self-care strengthen perseverance. Matthew 6:34 (AMP) teaches, *"So do not worry about tomorrow; for tomorrow will worry about itself. Each day has enough trouble of its own."* while Colossians 3:13 (AMP) reminds us, *"Bearing graciously with one another, and willingly forgiving each other if one has a cause for complaint against another; just as the Lord has forgiven you, so should you forgive."*

Deeper Reflection

Identify the community you have or the community you desire. What does it look like? How does it make you feel?

Assignment

Reach out to one person in your community to share encouragement or seek support.

Day 48:

Applying Mental Toughness & Resilience

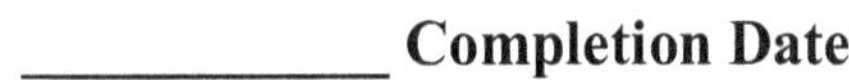 **Completion Date**

As we have studied, mental toughness combines discipline, resilience, and spiritual grounding. Challenges may arise in crises, as Job or Naomi experienced, or in mundane routines. Using prayer, Scripture, community, self-care, and reflection allows us to maintain consistency, overcome setbacks, and keep progressing toward goals. Joshua 1:9 (AMP) reminds us, *"Have I not commanded you? Be strong and courageous! Do not be terrified or dismayed (intimidated), for the Lord your God is with you wherever you go."* Romans 8:28 (AMP) reassures us, *"And we know [with great confidence] that God [who is deeply concerned about us] causes all things to work together [as a plan] for good for those who love God, to those who are called according to His plan and purpose."*

Deeper Reflection

1. How can you integrate mental toughness and spiritual tools into your daily routine?

2. Which strategies will you prioritize during challenging or mundane times?

Day 49:
Recognizing Strength in the Mundane

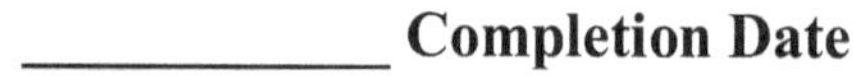

____________ Completion Date

Mental strength is built in ordinary moments—the quiet adherence to a daily routine, choosing faith over frustration, or responding with patience. Mundane days shape character and resilience. Job trusted God despite loss, and Jonah obeyed God's calling despite personal reluctance. Psalm 127:1 (AMP) reminds us, *"Unless the Lord builds the house, They labor in vain who build it; Unless the Lord guards the city, The watchman keeps awake in vain."*

Deeper Reflection

1. What ordinary routines or habits help you maintain mental and spiritual resilience in the mundane?

2. How can you infuse intentionality into mundane daily tasks?

3. In what ways can you reflect on your progress to see the impact of consistent effort?

Day 50:
Leaning on Community and Scripture

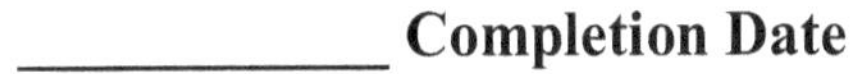 **Completion Date**

No one was meant to walk life alone. Community provides accountability, encouragement, and perspective. Scripture reminds us that "two are better than one" because we are strengthened through shared effort and mutual support (Ecclesiastes 4:9–12, AMP). Just as Naomi leaned on Ruth, your spiritual and mental foundation is strengthened through connection with others who uplift you, help you stand when you stumble, and remind you of truth when you feel weary.

Deeper Reflection

1. Who in your community can you lean on for accountability and encouragement?

2. How does Scripture help you navigate challenges or discouragement?

Days 1 to 50:

Dig Deeper Day

____________ **Completion Date**

Pause & Review

This is not a reset—it's a reminder of how far you've come and where God is still leading. Each day you've completed is not a checkmark of completion but another layer added to your lifelong healthy foundation in God.

On this day, pause and look back over all the work you've done so far. Notice the patterns God is weaving, the lessons that repeat, and the areas where your strength and faith are growing. Take time to adjust, change, and update your responses as you feel led—this is a journey of ongoing refinement.

Helpful Reflection Prompts

1. What have I learned about God through my journey so far?

2. How have I seen growth in my body, mind, and spirit from Day 1 until now?

3. What themes or lessons keep resurfacing, showing me where God is calling me to go deeper?

4. What practices or insights do I want to carry with me into the next stage of the journey?

Day 51:
Mental Toughness Through Scripture (Revisited)

_____________ Completion Date

Mental toughness isn't just enduring hardships—it's responding with faith, perseverance, and intentionality. Jonah shows that even when we resist God's plan, His guidance redirects us (Jonah 1:1-17). Job endured suffering, yet trusted God's sovereignty and experienced restoration (Job 1:20-22; 42:10-17). Psalm 34:17-19 (AMP) reminds us, *"The righteous cry out, and the Lord hears them; he delivers them from all their troubles. The Lord is close to the brokenhearted and saves those who are crushed in spirit."*

Deeper Reflection

How can you intentionally respond with faith when faced with discouragement or setbacks?

Day 52:
Creating Your Personal Disaster Plan

_______________ **Completion Date**

Life will not always go smoothly. Even small disruptions can test resilience. Just as we plan for emergencies, we can create a "disaster plan" for mental and spiritual well-being. Identify strategies and Scripture passages to lean on when life becomes difficult. As a reminder, Philippians 4:6-7 (AMP) reminds us, *"Do not be anxious or worried about anything, but in everything [every circumstance and situation] by prayer and petition with thanksgiving, continue to make your [specific] requests known to God. And the peace of God [that peace which reassures the heart, that peace] which transcends all understanding, stands guard over your hearts and your minds in Christ Jesus."*

There is strength and comfort in knowing what to do when life goes off course—because it will. Difficulty does not mean failure; it means you are human in a broken world. Having a plan in place provides direction when emotions are high and clarity feels distant. Just as travelers learn landmarks to find their way back on the trail, we need familiar practices and truths to guide us when life feels disorienting.

Knowing your way back matters. In the wilderness seasons of life, Scripture, prayer, and intentional response become your compass. They remind you who you are, where your help comes from, and how to take the next faithful step forward—even when the path feels unclear.

Deeper Reflection

1. What practical tools or practices can you include in your disaster plan?

2. Which Scripture passages provide comfort and guidance during challenges?

3. How can your disaster plan help you remain consistent in faith and mental resilience?

Assignment

• Write your personal disaster plan including prayers, Scripture, self-care, and support strategies. Place it somewhere meaningful and memorable to be easily accessible.

• Review it weekly and adjust as needed for ongoing resilience.

Day 53:

Gratitude and Reflection as Strength

_________ **Completion Date**

Using gratitude to build mental and spiritual resilience. Gratitude is a powerful tool for mental strength. Reflecting on your blessings shifts your focus from what is missing to what God has provided. Just as charted progress highlights milestones and small victories, gratitude helps you recognize daily growth.

As a refresher, 1 Thessalonians 5:16-18 (AMP) reminds us, _"Rejoice always and delight in your faith; be unceasing and persistent in prayer; in every situation [no matter what the circumstances] be thankful and continually give thanks to God; for this is the will of God for you in Christ Jesus."_ By intentionally practicing gratitude, you cultivate a mindset that is resilient in the face of adversity and grounded in God's faithfulness. Even on mundane days, listing your blessings and noting God's presence strengthens your spiritual foundation.

Deeper Reflection

1. What are three things you can thank God for today?

2. How does gratitude shift your perspective during challenges or monotony?

3. How can you integrate daily gratitude into your ongoing spiritual practice?

Day 54:
Continuing the Journey

____________ Completion Date

As you continue on, remember that your God-centered foundation requires ongoing care. Just like a potter lovingly caring for their work in the many stages of creation, God does everything for our consideration.

Remember Jonah's redemption, Job's perseverance, and Naomi's hope as reminders that God sustains and restores even when life seems unpredictable (Jonah 3:1-10; Job 42:10-17; Ruth 1:16-18). Philippians 4:13 (AMP) encourages us: *"I can do all things [which He has called me to do] through Him who strengthens and empowers me [to fulfill His purpose—I am self-sufficient in Christ's sufficiency]; I am ready for anything and equal to anything through Him who infuses me with inner strength and confident peace."* You have developed tools of mental toughness, self-discipline, gratitude, and reliance on Scripture that will serve you in daily life. Continue to lean into prayer, community, and reflection to protect and nourish your foundation.

Deeper Reflection

1. How will you ensure your journey receives on-going care?

2. How can you support others in their journey while maintaining your own growth?

Day 55:
Fortitude in Small Choices

____________ **Completion Date**

Life is not defined by a single mistake, nor is growth defined by a single success. Just as making one poor choice does not determine your life, making one good choice does not instantly resolve all challenges—but it does build fortitude over time. Every intentional step, no matter how small, is part of the harvest God has promised for perseverance.

As a refresher, Galatians 6:9 (AMP) reminds us: *"Let us not grow weary or become discouraged in doing good, for at the proper time we will reap, if we do not give in."*

Fortitude is cultivated in everyday decisions—choosing integrity when no one is watching, showing kindness when it's inconvenient, or staying faithful to your goals even when results are slow. Think of it like planting seeds: a single seed doesn't sprout overnight. But careful, consistent planting, watering, and tending leads to a fruitful harvest. Your persistence in doing what is right, even in small ways, strengthens character, reinforces discipline, and positions you for God's blessing.

Deeper Reflection

1. What small choices today can demonstrate fortitude in your life?

2. How do you remind yourself that one action doesn't define your journey?

3. Which areas in your life require consistency to see God's "harvest"?

Day 56:
Bearing Good Fruit

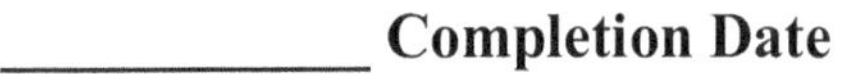 **Completion Date**

Our lives are a reflection of what we produce. God measures our hearts and actions by the fruit we bear. What we produce is shaped by what we consistently give our attention to, invest our time in, and choose to practice each day. Like a fruit tree, fruit takes time, patience, and care — but it will show what has been nurtured within.

Picture a fig tree. At first, it is just a small sapling, then buds appear, and eventually, the fruit begins to grow. It doesn't happen overnight. The tree must be rooted, nourished, and tended patiently. Even in the winter, when the trees appear lifeless, they are resting and preparing for spring.

When I began dating my husband, it was the middle of winter, and we often drove through the old orchards in his hometown. I remember commenting on how all the trees looked dead—pruned back, curled bare branches, and lifeless. He laughed and gently corrected me. "They're not dead," he said. "They're dormant."

Your life is like that tree. Every choice, word, and action contributes to the kind of fruit you produce. Sometimes it feels like nothing is changing, but God is at work, shaping your character and cultivating your heart. Judgement on fruit is not instantaneous — it comes at harvest. Good fruit reflects kindness, patience, love, joy, and integrity. Just as a tree doesn't grow fruit in isolation, your life needs the nourishment of God's Word, prayer, and spiritual discipline.

Deeper Reflection

1. What "fruit" is currently evident in your life?

2. Are there areas where you feel God is still cultivating growth?

3. How can you nurture the fruit in your life intentionally each day?

Assignment

Create a piece of fruit—using clay, paper, or another creative medium—that represents your spiritual growth or the qualities you want to cultivate. On or inside the fruit, write or symbolize the qualities you are intentionally growing: patience, faith, love, gratitude, etc. Display it somewhere visible as a reminder of God's work in you and the patience required to bear good fruit.

Day 57:

Bedrock: Reviewing Your Foundation

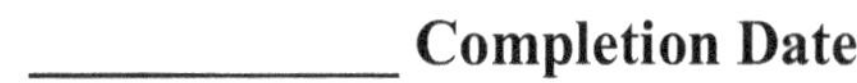

______________ **Completion Date**

Before building new layers in your life, pause to take stock of your foundation: gratitude practices, reflection routines, and intentional focus on small daily choices. These are your "bricks and mortar." They may seem simple, but they form the solid ground that will hold everything else you build.

Review your journal entries and notes from the previous weeks. Reflect on the lessons that resonated most.

Romans 12:1 (AMP) reminds us: *"Therefore I urge you, brothers and sisters, by the mercies of God, to present your bodies [dedicating all of yourselves, set apart] as a living sacrifice, holy and well-pleasing to God, which is your rational (logical, intelligent) act of worship."*

Deeply reflect on the progress you've made so far.

Deeper Reflection

1. Which lessons from your journey so far resonate most with you?

2. Which habits feel strong, and which ones need to be reinforced?

Day 58:
Anchoring in Awareness

_______________ **Completion Date**

Awareness is the quiet superpower of transformation. Being mindful of your body, thoughts, emotions, and daily choices allows you to see patterns clearly and adjust before old habits take hold.

Pay attention to your meals, energy levels, interactions, and daily routines. Awareness helps you make intentional changes that align with your health, goals, and faith. Proverbs 4:7 (AMP) reminds us: *"The beginning of wisdom is: Get [skillful and godly] wisdom [it is preeminent]! And with all your acquiring, get understanding [actively seek spiritual discernment, mature comprehension, and logical interpretation]."*

In pottery, awareness is learned in the quiet stages—especially during the drying process. Clay does not dry all at once, and the changes are subtle. To an untrained eye, nothing appears to be happening, but a skilled potter knows exactly what to look for: shifts in color, temperature, firmness, and tension. These small cues tell you when to slow down, when to cover the piece, when to uncover it, and when to wait. Ignoring these signs can lead to cracking, warping, or collapse.

Learning to notice these subtle changes is what moves a pottery student toward mastery. The clay teaches you to pay attention, to respond rather than rush, and to adjust before damage occurs. In the same way, developing awareness in your body, mind, and spirit allows you to recognize patterns early and make course corrections before old habits harden. Awareness becomes the quiet discipline that protects growth and supports lasting transformation.

Deeper Reflection

1. What patterns have you observed in your daily habits, nutrition, or mindset?

2. How can increased awareness guide you to make intentional, positive changes?

3. What small adjustment can you implement today based on your observations?

4. Write down one pattern you've noticed in your health, mindset, or daily habits. Reflect on how increased awareness might help you course-correct or reinforce positive behaviors. This reflection strengthens your ability to act intentionally and maintain consistency in growth.

Day 59:
Gratitude in Action

______________ **Completion Date**

Gratitude is more than a feeling—it's a practice. Actively noticing and appreciating small blessings—health, meals, strength, and loved ones—shifts your mindset and strengthens resilience.

Active gratitude reinforces your spiritual foundation and nurtures mindfulness in everyday life.

Choosing active gratitude shapes your habits, responses to challenges, and your perspective on daily routines. Integrating gratitude into your daily practice creates a mindset that remains resilient in both ordinary and difficult moments.

Deeper Reflection

1. What are three things you are grateful for today?

2. How does recognizing these blessings influence your daily habits and choices?

3. How can you incorporate more intentional gratitude?

Day 60:

The Power of Small Choices (Revisited)

__________ **Completion Date**

We have studied that transformation doesn't happen in giant leaps—it happens in consistent, small steps. Each choice you make—what you eat, how you move, how you speak to yourself—is a building block toward the life God intends for you. Even seemingly minor decisions contribute to the harvest of discipline, perseverance, and spiritual growth.

As a refresher, Galatians 6:9 (AMP) reminds us: *"Let us not grow weary or become discouraged in doing good, for at the proper time we will reap, if we do not give in."*

Take a moment today to notice the small choices before you. Reflect on how intentionally selecting what aligns with your health, habits, and faith contributes to your growth. Each step matters, and God honors your faithful attention to even the smallest actions.

Deeper Reflection

- What three small choices can I make today that align with my health and spiritual goals?
- How can I stay mindful throughout the day to ensure these choices are intentional?

Days 1 to 60:

Dig Deeper Day

_________________ **Completion Date**

Pause & Review

This is not a reset—it's a reminder of how far you've come and where God is still leading. Each day you've completed is not a checkmark of completion but another layer added to your lifelong healthy foundation in God.

On this day, pause and look back over all the work you've done so far. Notice the patterns God is weaving, the lessons that repeat, and the areas where your strength and faith are growing. Take time to adjust, change, and update your responses as you feel led—this is a journey of ongoing refinement.

Helpful Reflection Prompts

1. What have I learned about God through my journey so far?

2. How have I seen growth in my body, mind, and spirit from Day 1 until now?

3. What themes or lessons keep resurfacing, showing me where God is calling me to go deeper?

4. What practices or insights do I want to carry with me into the next stage of the journey?

Day 61:
Building Focus

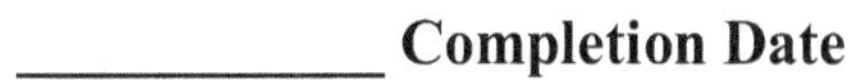

Completion Date

Focus is the lens through which habits gain meaning. Cultivate it through mindful attention to your movements, meals, prayers, and daily tasks. When distractions arise, gently bring yourself back to the task at hand. Focus allows you to honor God by fully engaging with the present moment and the work He has set before you.

Focus does not require rigidity. Life does not happen in a vacuum. Plans shift, interruptions arise, or energy is limited. Giving yourself permission to adjust without abandoning your intention is part of faithful focus. Choose presence over perfection. This allows you to stay engaged rather than discouraged. When you respond to life with grace and adaptability, focus becomes a practice you return to—not a standard you fail.

Reflection Questions

- Reflect on one area of your day where you can practice intentional focus—whether in a workout, meal preparation, or a time of prayer. Notice how undivided attention transforms not only your productivity but also your connection to God and the discipline of your mind.

- Which part of your day can benefit most from intentional focus?

- What distractions commonly pull you away, and how can you redirect yourself?

- How does cultivating focus strengthen your spiritual, mental, and physical growth?

Day 62:
Faith in Your Progress

_____________ **Completion Date**

Faith is the quiet belief that your efforts are not in vain, even when results are not immediately visible. Trusting God's timing and your ability to grow allows patience and perseverance to take root. Faith gives perspective, reminding you that transformation is often unseen until harvest.

Hebrews 11:1 (AMP) teaches: *"Now faith is the assurance (title deed, confirmation) of things hoped for (divinely guaranteed), and the evidence of things not seen [the conviction of their reality—faith comprehends as fact what cannot be experienced by the physical senses]."*

I remember being in my pottery studio in the early years, walking from one room to another, when something suddenly stopped me. As I looked around, I realized I was standing in the middle of prayers God had already answered—prayers I had given, not knowing how or when He would respond. I had been living inside those answers without even recognizing them.

The realization was overwhelming. I dropped to my knees, sobbing—not from sorrow, but from awe and deep gratitude. I was undone by His faithfulness. God had been working quietly, steadily, and faithfully all along, even when I could not yet see it. That moment forever changed how I understand faith: not as blind hope, but as trust in a God who is always at work, often far beyond what we notice in the day-to-day.

Reflection Questions

- Take time today to reflect on recent successes or breakthroughs in your journey. Consider the role faith has played in making those moments possible, and how trusting God in the unseen strengthens your resolve to continue.
- How has faith supported my progress even when I didn't see immediate results?
- What recent breakthrough can I thank God for?
- How can I nurture faith in my daily choices moving forward?

Day 63:
Self-Care as Discipline

_________________ **Completion Date**

Self-care is often expressed through small, ordinary acts done consistently. Simple routines like basic hygiene, skincare, nourishing meals, regular movement, adequate sleep, and caring for your physical environment all contribute to how you feel and function each day. These practices are not about vanity or perfection; they are about respect for the body God designed and entrusted to you.

When these small acts are approached with intention, they become anchors in daily life. A workout becomes a way to steward strength. Hygiene and personal care become moments of dignity and presence. Rest becomes an act of trust. Over time, these seemingly simple choices compound, supporting resilience, clarity, and readiness to show up fully for what God has called you to do.

Reflection Questions

• Take a moment to identify one self-care practice that recharges your spirit and supports your physical and mental health. Commit to practicing it intentionally today, noticing how it strengthens your ability to show up faithfully for yourself and others.

• Which self-care practice today will most support my health and spiritual growth?

• How does consistent self-care contribute to discipline and resilience?

• How can I integrate this practice into my daily routine without guilt or distraction?

Day 64:

Sustaining Growth Through Reflection

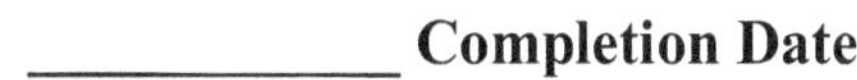

_________________ **Completion Date**

Reflection solidifies progress. Pausing to consider lessons learned, patterns noticed, and victories celebrated keeps your foundation strong. It allows you to adjust, reinforce, and continue growing intentionally.

Lamentations 3:40 (AMP) reminds us: *"Let us test and examine our ways, And let us return to the Lord."* Reflection helps you stay aligned with God's purpose and reinforces mental, spiritual, and physical resilience.

Reflection Questions

• Take time today to review your recent progress. What worked well? What requires adjustment? How does God's presence guide your next steps?

• What recent actions or habits have had the greatest positive impact on my growth?

• How can reflection deepen my connection with God and strengthen my consistency?

Day 65:
Continuing the Foundation

____________ Completion Date

As you continue, remember the lessons from the previous days. Each intentional practice of gratitude, faith, and discipline strengthens what has already been laid. Growth often happens in places we would rather avoid—the uncomfortable moments, the challenges, and the situations that stretch us beyond what feels familiar.

God equips you with what you need to keep building: self-control, prayer, reflection, and steady obedience. When discomfort arises, allow it to deepen your reliance on Him rather than derail your progress. Each faithful choice—no matter how small—adds another layer of strength to your spiritual, mental, and physical foundation, preparing you to endure and grow with resilience.

Reflection Questions

Which tools am I using consistently to strengthen my foundation?

Day 66:
Put It Away, Don't Put It Down (Revisited)

_____________ **Completion Date**

"Put it away—don't put it down" (PIA-DPID) is an exercise trains self-control and discipline in small, everyday moments. It could be putting your hairbrush back in the drawer, washing dishes immediately, or putting laundry away. These actions seem insignificant on their own, but they build something much bigger beneath the surface.

Each time you choose to complete a task fully, you reinforce follow-through, order, and intentionality. Over time, these small decisions begin to shape your mindset. You start trusting yourself more. Your environment becomes calmer and more supportive. Discipline practiced in these quiet moments spill into larger areas of life—how you eat, how you move, how you manage time, how you respond under stress. What begins as a simple habit becomes a pattern of obedience and consistency that strengthens your foundation far beyond the task itself.

Deeper Reflection

Discipline is often tested in the ordinary, unseen choices. How you manage small responsibilities reflects your readiness for bigger ones. These everyday victories prepare your heart for greater faithfulness.

• Reflect on how small acts of discipline in your daily routine shape larger habits.

- Notice whether order in your environment creates greater peace in your heart.
- Consider how faithfulness in these little actions builds spiritual maturity.

Verse for Study

1 Corinthians 14:40 (AMP): *"But all things must be done appropriately and in an orderly manner."*

Day 67:
Understanding Discipline

_________________ **Completion Date**

Discipline is more than following rules—it's a virtue allowing you to exercise self-control. Through intentional self-control, you strengthen not just your habits, but your character, faith, and ability to serve others. Discipline is empowerment, not punishment.

Self-control is the pause that creates space for discipline to take shape. It is the moment of stopping, noticing, and processing before a decision is made. In that pause, you are given the opportunity to choose wisely rather than react automatically. Discipline grows when self-control is practiced repeatedly in these small moments—choosing alignment over impulse, intention over habit. This pause is not weakness; it is strength exercised quietly, allowing faith, wisdom, and purpose to guide the next step.

Deeper Reflection

- Discipline is not about restriction—it is about direction. God uses discipline to refine, strengthen, and align your steps with His purpose. It brings freedom rather than bondage.
- Reflect on how discipline brings freedom rather than restriction.
- Recall a moment when exercising discipline helped you grow spiritually or physically.

Verse for Study

Hebrews 12:11 (AMP): *"For the time being no discipline*

brings joy, but seems sad and painful; yet to those who have been trained by it, afterwards it yields the peaceful fruit of righteousness [right standing with God and a lifestyle and attitude that seeks conformity to God's will and purpose]."

Day 68:
Embracing the Uncomfortable

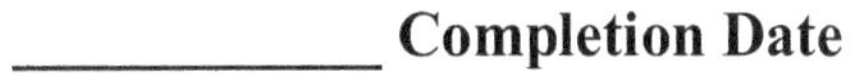

_________ Completion Date

Growth requires discomfort. You've already begun by showing up for this journey, even without knowing all the details.

Comfort zones feel safe, but they rarely produce growth. God stretches you through challenges, allowing discomfort to become a place where perseverance, trust, and resilience are built.

Deeper Reflection

Today's focus is identifying areas where you can push beyond comfort.

- Reflect on why stepping into discomfort can be an act of faith.
- Consider the spiritual strength you've already gained through challenges.
- Identify one place in life where God may be calling you to go further.

Verse for Study

James 1:3 (AMP): *"Be assured that the testing of your faith [through experience] produces endurance [leading to spiritual maturity, and inner peace]."*

Day 69:
Writing a Prayer of Discipline

________________ **Completion Date**

Spiritual discipline through prayer acknowledges reliance on God while committing to growth in self-control and virtue. Prayer is both surrender and strength. By bringing your desire for discipline before God, you invite His Spirit to guide your thoughts, habits, and words into alignment with His will.

Deeper Reflection

- Write your own prayer of discipline, asking God for strength in self-control, the precursor to self-discipline.
- Reflect on how prayer deepens your discipline and strengthens your walk. Place the prayer somewhere visible and meaningful.
- Consider what area of your life you need to surrender most to God's Spirit.

Verse for Study

Psalm 141:3 (AMP): *"Set a guard, O Lord, over my mouth; Keep watch over the door of my lips [to keep me from speaking thoughtlessly]."*

Day 70:
Faithfulness in the Small Things (Revisited)

__________ **Completion Date**

Faithfulness in the little things reflects faithfulness in the big things. By practicing discipline in small acts—putting things away, completing minor tasks—you train yourself to handle greater responsibilities.

Deeper Reflection

Small acts of obedience are not wasted. Each one is a seed of trust, proving your faithfulness and opening the door for God to entrust you with more.

- Reflect on how God honors small steps of obedience.
- Consider which "little things" in your life need greater attention.

Days 1 to 70:
Dig Deeper Day

_____________ **Completion Date**

Pause & Review

This is not a reset—it's a reminder of how far you've come and where God is still leading. Each day you've completed is not a checkmark of completion but another layer added to your lifelong healthy foundation in God.

On this day, pause and look back over all the work you've done so far. Notice the patterns God is weaving, the lessons that repeat, and the areas where your strength and faith are growing. Take time to adjust, change, and update your responses as you feel led—this is a journey of ongoing refinement.

Helpful Reflection Prompts

1. What have I learned about God through my journey so far?

2. How have I seen growth in my body, mind, and spirit from Day 1 until now?

3. What themes or lessons keep resurfacing, showing me where God is calling me to go deeper?

4. What practices or insights do I want to carry with me into the next stage of the journey?

Day 71:
Stop Listening to the Noise (Revisited)

_______________ **Completion Date**

There is a lot of conflicting information about health, fitness, and nutrition—it can be overwhelming. We need to be mindful and continue to identify the noise and intentionally filter it out.

Noise pulls us away from God's truth and the simple, steady disciplines that bring long-term growth. What seems shiny and promising in the moment usually distracts us from lasting habits and from trusting God's design for our bodies. Filtering out the noise helps us focus on what really matters—faith, consistency, and the small steps that honor Him.

Deeper Reflection

- Identify at least one example of "noise" you've noticed recently (fad diet, supplement, gimmick, or quick fix).
- Write down why it won't work long-term.
- Reflect on how your foundation in faith, self-control, and focus can guide you away from distractions.

Verse for Study

Proverbs 4:25 (AMP): *"Let your eyes look directly ahead [toward the path of moral courage],And let your gaze be fixed straight in front of you [toward the path of integrity]."*

Day 72:
Hope, Planning, and Grace

__________ **Completion Date**

Even as you plan your life, remember: we are never promised tomorrow. Life is uncertain, but we can live with hope and purpose today. Planning matters, but our hope rests not in our schedules or perfect execution, but in God's grace and strength.

Sometimes our desire for control can creep into health goals, making us strive in pride rather than rest in God's grace. Hope and humility remind us that God is in charge of the outcome, and our role is obedience and faithfulness in the small steps.

Deeper Reflection

- Journal about how hope guides your health and fitness journey.
- Reflect on how humility changes the way you approach your daily choices.
- Write one way you can show grace to yourself if your plan doesn't go perfectly this week.

Verse for Study

James 4:6 (AMP): *"But He gives us more and more grace [through the power of the Holy Spirit to defy sin and live an obedient life that reflects both our faith and our gratitude for our salvation]. Therefore it says, 'God is opposed to the proud and haughty, but [continually] gives the gift of grace to the humble [who turn away from self-righteousness].'"*

Day 73:
Designed to Be Fueled

______________ Completion Date

Our bodies are not meant to be abused, starved, or overloaded—they are designed to be fueled. God created our bodies as intricate, resilient, and purposeful machines. Every cell, muscle, and organ relies on intentional nourishment to function, move, and serve His purpose. Fueling our body properly honors the Creator and allows us to walk in strength, clarity, and vitality.

Too often, the world teaches consumption for pleasure, convenience, or comfort. Mindless eating, bingeing, or following every fad diet can feel satisfying in the moment but ultimately works against our design. Instead, intentional fuel provides energy, supports recovery, and strengthens mental and spiritual focus. Think of your body like a high-performance tool: it performs best when maintained and nourished, not overused or neglected.

Deeper Reflection

- Reflect on how your current eating habits either fuel or consume your body.

- Consider one small change today that shifts your focus from consumption to intentional nourishment.

- How does viewing your body as God's designed temple change your choices in food, movement, and rest?

Verse for Study

1 Corinthians 6:19-20 (AMP): *"Do you not know that*

your body is a temple of the Holy Spirit who is within you, whom you have [received as a gift] from God, and that you are not your own [property]? You were bought with a price [you were actually purchased with the precious blood of Jesus and made His own]. So then, honor and glorify God with your body."

Day 74:
Designed to Move

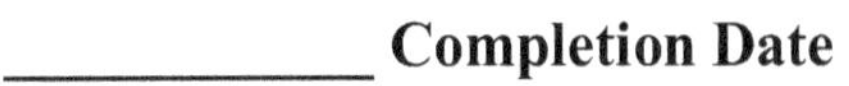

_________ Completion Date

God created our bodies to move. Movement is not optional—it is part of our design. Every joint, muscle, and bone functions best when active, whether through walking, stretching, lifting, or simply being intentional with posture. Movement supports circulation, mental clarity, emotional health, and spiritual focus. It allows us to fully engage in life and serve God with strength and vitality.

Too often, modern life encourages prolonged sitting, passivity, and convenience over intentional activity. When we neglect movement, our bodies become sluggish, our energy wanes, and our health suffers. But when we move with purpose, honoring God in every step, we cultivate discipline, resilience, and joy in our bodies. Movement is worship in motion—it reflects gratitude for the gift of a body that can act, serve, and glorify God.

Deeper Reflection

- Reflect on your daily movement: how much of it is intentional versus incidental?
- Identify one type of movement you can commit to today that honors your body and God's design.
- Consider how regular movement impacts not just your physical health, but your mental clarity, emotional resilience, and spiritual focus.

Verse for Study

1 Timothy 4:8 (AMP): *"For physical training is of some value (useful for a little), but godliness [spiritual training] is useful and of value in everything and in every way, since it holds promise for the present life and for the life to come."*

Day 75:
Movement & Nutrition

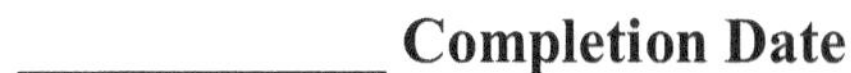

__________ Completion Date

Remembering that the view of a healthy lifestyle is going to look different for everyone. However, we are all designed to be fueled and to move. With that in mind…when I first began rebuilding my health, my steps were small. I didn't start with heavy workouts or complicated programs. I began with movement I could manage—yoga-inspired stretches like the cobra pose to strengthen my spine and restore mobility. These daily practices became more than exercise; they were a reminder that faithfulness in the small things matters.

Movement also taught me discipline. Just as feeding my body with nourishing food supported healing, consistent stretching and exercise trained not only my muscles but also my heart and mind to stay focused. Over time, I learned that strength is built little by little, and God multiplies the results when we show up faithfully.

You don't need a perfect workout plan to see progress. You need intentionality and consistency. Every time you move your body, you're stewarding the temple God entrusted to you. Think of your health journey as planting seeds—movement and nutrition are the daily watering, and in time, God brings growth.

Deeper Reflection

- Write down one small movement routine you can commit to this week (it might be stretching, a short walk, or simple bodyweight exercises).

- Reflect on how proper nutrition and movement together can create lasting health.
- Consider how building consistency in movement mirrors building consistency in prayer and time with God.

Verse for Study

1 Corinthians 9:27 (AMP): *"But [like a boxer] I strictly discipline my body and make it my slave, so that, after I have preached [the Good News] to others, I myself will not somehow be disqualified [as unfit for service]."*

Day 76:
The Gym

Once I felt ready, I joined a gym. At first, it wasn't about lifting heavy or mastering every machine—it was about learning, showing up, and becoming comfortable in a new environment. The gym gave me space to grow, but I also paid attention to the nudges of the Holy Spirit. Over time, I felt Him closing that chapter and guiding me toward building a small, mindful home gym. That shift reminded me: our health journey isn't one-size-fits-all. God directs each of us differently.

The gym—whether public or at home—isn't just about equipment. It's a training ground for discipline. Some days you'll feel motivated, but many days you won't. That's when self-control and perseverance matter most. We aren't just training muscles—we're training our minds and spirits to stay steady in obedience.

Equally important is what we put into our bodies. You can never out-train poor nutrition. The world bombards us with convenience foods and fad diets, but true fuel looks different. For me, I've found a macro-based approach works best. It allows for balance—fats, proteins, and carbs in the right proportions—without falling into extremes or gimmicks. Renewing our minds means rejecting the quick fixes the world offers and learning instead to steward our nutrition with wisdom and patience.

Deeper Reflection

Your body is God's temple, and both movement and nutrition are acts of worship. Don't compare your chapter one to someone else's chapter ten. Be faithful with what's in front of you today.

• Explore your gym or home workout options and note what feels sustainable and enjoyable for you.

• Remember—not every day will feel enjoyable. Reflect on how self-control and discipline play into showing up anyway.

• Consider how your choices in food mirror your choices in training: both require consistency, intention, and surrender to God's guidance.

Day 77:
Using a Trainer and Resources

__________ **Completion Date**

No one grows alone. Whether in faith, fitness, or daily life, God often strengthens us through the wisdom, support, and accountability of others. Using a trainer, coach, mentor, or resource isn't a sign of weakness — it's evidence of humility and teachability. It means you recognize that growth is not meant to be isolated; it's meant to be supported.

Just like in spiritual growth, there are moments in where you need someone who sees your blind spots, encourages your potential, and helps you stay consistent. A trainer can teach proper form, prevent injury, and bring clarity to your goals. Spiritually, the Holy Spirit does the same — guiding, correcting, strengthening, and leading you into deeper truth. When you invite guidance into your journey, you honor God by acknowledging that you cannot do this alone.

Using resources — workout plans, videos, nutrition tools, gym equipment, or community support — doesn't replace God's work in you; it helps you steward the body He entrusted to you. God will often use people and tools as part of your growth story. You aren't meant to figure everything out without help.

Today, let yourself be led, supported, and equipped. Growth is easier when you lean into the resources God has placed around you.

Deeper Reflection

- Where in your fitness journey do you need guidance,

support, or accountability?

• What resource or person might God be inviting you to lean into today?

• How can you practice humility by receiving help instead of carrying everything alone?

Verse for Study

Proverbs 19:20 (AMP): *"Listen to counsel, receive instruction, and accept correction, that you may be wise in the time to come."*

Day 78:
Envision Your Healthy Self (Revisited)

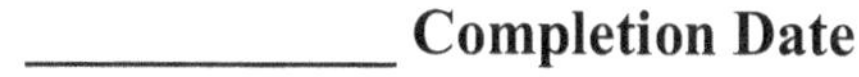

__________ **Completion Date**

Before anything becomes reality, it begins with vision. God often places a picture in your heart of **who you are becoming** — not to pressure you, but to guide you. Envisioning your healthy self is not about imagining perfection; it's about seeing the version of you who walks in alignment with God's truth, stewarding your body and soul with intention. It is important to revisit this growing version of yourself often.

This vision is meant to anchor you when you feel discouraged or stuck. When you picture your future self — stronger, more confident, more grounded, more surrendered — you reconnect with the purpose behind your daily choices. Vision is not fantasy. Vision is faith with direction.

Your healthy self is not someone far away. You are being built through every small choice — every walk, every nourishing meal, every moment of surrender, every prayer for strength, every time you come back after a rough day. When you envision yourself, you aren't pretending; you are agreeing with the work God is already doing.

Let this day be an invitation to look forward with hope, not pressure. You are growing into the version of you God designed — steadily, faithfully, with grace.

Deeper Reflection

- What qualities or habits do you picture when you imagine your healthiest, most grounded self?

• How is God already forming that version of you through small daily steps?

• What one action today aligns you with the person you are becoming?

Verse for Study

Habakkuk 2:2 (AMP): *"Write the vision and engrave it plainly... so that the one who reads it may run."*

Day 79:
Resilience, Intentionality, and Real Life

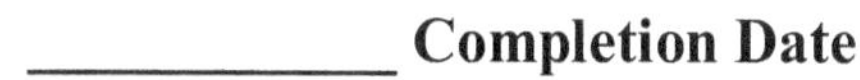

__________ **Completion Date**

Real life is messy, unpredictable, and rarely goes according to plan. But resilience is built not in perfect conditions — it's built in the middle of interruptions, setbacks, disappointments, and ordinary days. Your health journey is not exempt. You will have weeks where everything flows easily and weeks where nothing seems to align. Both matter. Both shape you.

Resilience isn't about always bouncing back instantly. It's about choosing, again and again, to stay connected to God and aligned with your purpose even when life feels heavy or busy. It's about returning to your foundation instead of abandoning it. Intentionality helps you make choices rooted in truth, not emotion. And God meets you in those choices — strengthening what is weak and steadying what feels unsteady.

When you practice resilience in your health, you are practicing spiritual endurance as well. You learn patience. You learn flexibility. You learn that progress is not linear. And you learn that God works in the imperfect, ordinary, unpolished parts of life just as much as the bright moments.

Days are not about perfection — it's about showing up with intention, trusting that God honors every small act of obedience.

Deeper Reflection
• Where is life feeling messy or unpredictable, and how can resilience show up there?

• What small intentional choice can you make today, even if the day feels imperfect?

• How have past challenges strengthened your current resilience?

Verse for Study

Galatians 6:9 (AMP): *"Let us not grow weary or become discouraged in doing good, for at the proper time we will reap, if we do not give in."*

Day 80:
On the Other Side
of Decisions

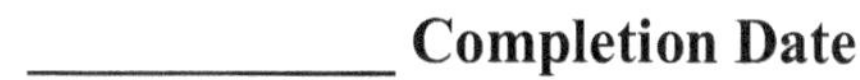

___________ **Completion Date**

Life decisions are rarely simple. They often hold layers of emotion, uncertainty, responsibility, and spiritual weight. Some decisions feel heavy because they touch your identity, your calling, your relationships, or your integrity. Others are difficult because they force you to confront fear, discomfort, or the possibility of disappointing someone you care about.

Recently, I faced a heart-wrenching decision. This choice was not made quickly or lightly. I prayed over it, wrestled with it, and felt the emotional weight of it. Yet walking through the process strengthened my resilience, deepened my trust in God, and reminded me that obedience sometimes asks us to release what once felt familiar.

On the other side of decisions—especially the difficult ones—you often find clarity you didn't have before. You see where God was nudging you. You sense where He was protecting you. You notice how He was shaping your character. Even when the outcome is painful or uncomfortable, making intentional decisions becomes an opportunity to grow in courage, integrity, and faith.

When your choices are aligned with your values, your purpose, and God's direction, you can move forward with peace, even if the path ahead is still unfolding. Decision-making becomes less about avoiding mistakes and more about trusting God to guide each step. You learn that you don't control the future—but you do control your obedience.

Whatever decision sits before you, large or small, God is already on the other side of it. You can move with intention, alignment, and a heart that desires His will above your comfort.

Deeper Reflection

• Reflect on a recent decision that required thought, prayer, or courage. What made it difficult or stretching?

• How did faith, Scripture, or the Holy Spirit guide your actions during the process?

• What clarity, lesson, or strengthening came *after* the decision was made?

• What fear or pressure tends to influence your decision-making? How can you invite God into that space?

• What upcoming decision could you approach with greater intention, surrender, or spiritual alignment?

Verse for Study

Proverbs 3:5–6 (AMP): *"Trust in and rely confidently on the Lord with all your heart and do not rely on your own insight or understanding. In all your ways know and acknowledge and recognize Him, and He will make your paths straight and smooth [removing obstacles that block your way]."*

Days 1 to 80:

Dig Deeper Day

_____________ **Completion Date**

Pause & Review

This is not a reset—it's a reminder of how far you've come and where God is still leading. Each day you've completed is not a checkmark of completion but another layer added to your lifelong healthy foundation in God.

On this day, pause and look back over all the work you've done so far. Notice the patterns God is weaving, the lessons that repeat, and the areas where your strength and faith are growing. Take time to adjust, change, and update your responses as you feel led—this is a journey of ongoing refinement.

Helpful Reflection Prompts

1. What have I learned about God through my journey so far?

2. How have I seen growth in my body, mind, and spirit from Day 1 until now?

3. What themes or lessons keep resurfacing, showing me where God is calling me to go deeper?

4. What practices or insights do I want to carry with me into the next stage of the journey?

Day 81:
Authenticity &
Transformation

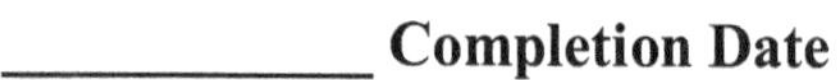 **Completion Date**

Transformation is not about becoming someone new — it's about becoming who God designed you to be. Authenticity and transformation work hand in hand. When you live honestly before God, without hiding or striving, you create space for true change to take root. God isn't asking for a polished version of you; He's asking for the real you — your fears, your hopes, your habits, your weaknesses, your desires.

Authenticity frees you to grow without pretending. It allows you to reflect on what is working, what isn't, and what God is inviting you to release. Transformation is a slow, faithful unfolding — built on honesty, humility, and openness to the Holy Spirit's shaping hand. You don't transform by force; you transform by surrender.

When you choose to be authentic in your health journey — acknowledging your triggers, patterns, and victories — God aligns your heart with truth. You stop aiming for perfection and start aiming for alignment. And alignment brings lasting transformation.

Becoming healthier is not about image, pressure, or performance. It's about becoming more rooted in who God created you to be.

Deeper Reflection
- Where is God inviting you to be more authentic with

yourself?

• What part of your health journey needs more honesty and less pressure?

• How is God transforming you—not instantly, but gradually—as you surrender?

Verse for Study

Ephesians 4:23–24 (AMP): *"Be continually renewed in the spirit of your mind... and put on the new self [the regenerated and God-like nature] created in God's image."*

Day 82:
Intentional Living

___________ Completion Date

Intentional living means making choices deliberately, consciously, and on purpose. It's about aligning your actions with your values, faith, and God's calling—even when the path is difficult, uncomfortable, or painful. Living intentionally is not about perfection, but about consistent, purposeful steps toward growth, character, and obedience.

God invites us to be purposeful in all areas of life—our health, relationships, work, and spiritual disciplines. Each decision, no matter how small, can reflect intentionality and honor God. When you pause, reflect, and act with awareness, you create space for God to work through your choices.

As a reminder, Proverbs 16:3 (AMP) tells us to *"Commit your works to the Lord [submit and trust them to Him], And your plans will succeed [if you respond to His will and guidance]."*

Deeper Reflection

- Look up the definition of "intentional" and write it in your own words.
- Identify one example in the Bible of intentional living.
- Reflect on your week ahead: How can you live more intentionally in your health, relationships, and faith? What practical steps can you take today to act with purpose?

Day 83:
Strength Training Your Confidence

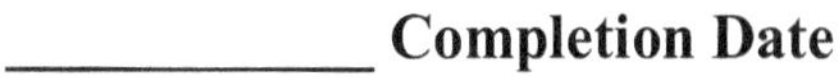

_____________ **Completion Date**

Confidence isn't something that appears suddenly; it develops gradually, the same way physical strength does. You don't begin with the heaviest weight. You begin with what your body and mind can carry, and as you show up consistently, you build the foundation for greater strength.

In the same way, internal strength — spiritual confidence — must be built before external transformation can truly take root. If the mind is still anchored in fear, comparison, excuses, or old patterns, physical progress cannot sustain itself. God invites you to begin inside first: renewing your mind, grounding your identity, aligning your choices with truth, and trusting His voice over your feelings.

Movement becomes a training ground, yes — but it is not the starting point. God starts the transformation in your mind and spirit, and fitness becomes one of the ways that transformation is lived out.

Today, tend your internal foundation. Confidence grows as you keep showing up with a willing heart, rooted in God's truth.

Deeper Reflection

• How has your mindset grown stronger throughout this journey?

• What internal belief is God reshaping as He strengthens

your confidence?

• What movement today can reflect the inner work God is already doing?

Verse for Study

Psalm 18:32 (AMP): *"It is God who arms me with strength and makes my way perfect."*

Day 84:
Movement as Worship

__________ **Completion Date**

Worship isn't limited to songs or quiet moments. Your daily movement can also become an offering to God — but that offering becomes meaningful when your heart and mind are aligned first. This devotional has guided you through the internal transformation necessary to view movement not as punishment or pressure, but as stewardship and gratitude.

God designed your body to move, but He calls you to begin the journey inside: renewing your mind, grounding your identity, and aligning your intentions. When you move with a renewed purpose — not to earn worth but to honor God — movement becomes worship. It's not about the routine you choose.

Movement doesn't need to be extreme to be worshipful. It simply needs to be intentional. When your inner foundation is strong, your physical choices become an extension of that strength. Let your movement today reflect your gratitude for the body God created and the transformation He is cultivating within you.

Deeper Reflection

- How does recognizing movement as worship shift your mindset?
- Where can you express gratitude through your body today?
- How does internal renewal shape the way you move physically?

Verse for Study

Romans 12:1 (AMP): *"Present your bodies... as a living sacrifice... your rational act of worship."*

Day 85:
Stepping Into a Healthier Calling

_____________ **Completion Date**

You have spent time renewing your mind, grounding your identity, and strengthening your spirit. This internal transformation is the root system that allows external transformation to grow and endure. Without this foundation, nutrition plans, movement routines, and healthy habits can crumble or return to old cycles. With this foundation, your choices become anchored in purpose instead of pressure.

Stepping into a healthier calling does not begin with performance—it begins with alignment. Alignment with God. Alignment with truth. Alignment with the person you are becoming. As your internal world strengthens, you will naturally make better decisions for your body: nourishment, steps, rest, movement, discipline, and stewardship. The sequence matters: Him → mindset → nourishment → movement. This is how your God-centered healthy lifestyle foundation is dug and your "house" is built on bedrock, not sand.

Deeper Reflection

- How is your internal transformation preparing you for sustainable physical change?
- What next step feels aligned with the person God is shaping you to be?
- How can you continue protecting and tending this foundation?

Verse for Study

Hebrews 12:1 (AMP): *"Let us run with endurance… the race that is set before us."*

Day 86:
Returning to Your Why

___________ **Completion Date**

Your "why" is the heartbeat of lasting transformation. It is the anchor that keeps you rooted when emotions shift, when discipline feels heavy, or when life tries to pull you off course. But your why must be renewed internally before it can fuel your physical transformation.

Many people begin with external goals, but this devotional has helped you do it God's way — starting with the internal work: truth, healing, identity, clarity, purpose, surrender, and mindset renewal. When your "why" is anchored in Christ, the steps you take toward nourishment, movement, and discipline will be stronger, steadier, and more sustainable.

Like envisioning your healthy self, returning to your why often is a core component to your God-centered foundation. Let it guide you. Let it ground you. Let it shape every choice you make next.

Deeper Reflection

• How has your why matured through internal transformation?

• What God-centered purpose now anchors your health journey?

• What aligned step is God inviting you to take next?

Verse for Study

Psalm 57:2 (AMP): *"He completes my purpose in His plan."*

Days 1 to 86:
Dig Deeper Day

____________ **Completion Date**

You've walked through 86 days of strengthening, nourishing, surrendering, building, and tending your God-centered healthy foundation. Today is not about adding more — it's about looking back with clarity and gratitude. God has been present in every choice, every challenge, every return, and every moment of growth. This day gives you space to breathe, reflect, and acknowledge the work He has done in your heart, mind, and body.

Use this day to slow down, revisit the lessons that shaped you most deeply, and allow God to speak into the next steps of your journey. This is not an ending — it is a moment of reflection, celebration, and alignment before walking forward with continued obedience and grace.

Deeper Reflection

• Which day or theme from Days 1–86 impacted you the most, and why?

• Where has God strengthened your foundation, and where is He inviting you to continue tending?

• What is one practice from this devotional you want to carry into your next season?

• How has your perspective on faith, health, and stewardship shifted throughout this journey?

Verse for Study

Philippians 1:6 (AMP): *"Being confident of this very*

thing, that He who began a good work in you will continue to perfect and complete it until the day of Christ Jesus."

Final Word & Commissioning

You've reached the culmination of this journey, and while the book may be ending, your transformation is only beginning. Over the past weeks, you have practiced surrender, discipline, and intentionality. You've strengthened your mind, aligned your actions with God-centered principles, and cultivated habits that support growth in every area of life.

Your life is like a river carving a canyon: consistent, purposeful flow shapes the landscape over time, creating depth and resilience you cannot achieve in a single day. Each choice you make, every intentional action, and each moment you devote to prayer, gratitude, and reflection builds the life God is calling you to live.

As you step into this next chapter, carry these truths with you:

- **Vision Beyond the Present** – Consider not just who you are today, but who you are becoming spiritually, mentally, and physically. Write your vision clearly, and revisit it often.
- **Empowered Choices** – Life is full of decisions. Choosing daily to act in alignment with faith, self-control, and discipline turns ordinary moments into milestones of transformation.
- **Faith in Motion** – Faith isn't passive. It is lived out in action. Applying what you've learned—through movement, reflection, service, and care for your body—turns intention into reality.

Take Time to Reflect
- What new daily habits will stretch your faith and dis-

cipline in the coming weeks?

- How can recent challenges become stepping stones rather than stumbling blocks?
- In what ways will the small, consistent actions you take today shape the life God is calling you to live?

Remember, your foundation is strong. You have practiced resilience, aligned your heart with God's purposes, and built habits that support lasting transformation. Step forward boldly, knowing that each intentional action, no matter how small, moves you closer to the abundant life God has prepared for you. Seek Him daily, apply His Word, and walk in confidence, knowing He is shaping your journey. As a reminder, Jeremiah 29:11 (AMP) tells us, *"For I know the plans and thoughts that I have for you," says the Lord, "plans for peace and well-being and not for disaster, to give you a future and a hope."*

Your journey continues beyond these pages. Each day is an opportunity to act, to grow, and to live intentionally for God's glory.

As you close this book, remember: this journey was never about perfection. It has always been about progress — faithful, steady, Spirit-led progress. The goal was not to arrive at a flawless finish line, but to build a God-centered healthy foundation you can continue to grow from day by day. Old strongholds break when the heart is surrendered, not when the habits are perfect.

Over this time together, you have stretched, listened, reflected, surrendered, and strengthened both your spirit and your body. Weather it took you 86 days or 86 weeks, you have learned to anchor your choices in God's truth, to steward your health with intention, and to let grace lead you instead of pressure. These days are not an ending — they are a beginning. A beginning of living with deeper awareness, clearer purpose, renewed thinking, and more grounded trust in the One who walks beside you.

The healthier we are — mentally, spiritually, and physically — the better we can serve God's purpose for our lives and serve others. That has always been the heartbeat of The Bodybuilding Potter. This journey is bigger than macros, movement, or mindset. It is about becoming the vessel God designed you to be: strengthened, refined, obedient, and available.

As you continue forward, remember that transformation begins internally and then expresses itself externally. Keep renewing your mind. Keep inviting God into your choices. When your heart stays aligned with Him, your nourishment, steps, movement, and discipline will naturally follow. And as you step deeper into this healthier calling, you do not have to walk alone.

I encourage you to stay engaged and connected. Share what God is doing in your life. Encourage someone else who needs hope. Continue building rhythms that honor God with your thoughts, your actions, and your body. Let your life be a light — a living testimony of God's grace at work in real time.

Together, we are a community seeking God's best — pursuing wholeness and holiness with intentionality and joy. As you go forward, may God strengthen your hands, steady your steps, and continue shaping you into the person He designed you to be.

You are loved.

You are called.

You are being formed by Him, the Master Potter.

Keep walking in His strength.

Closing Prayer of Commissioning

Heavenly Father, I lift up this reader into Your care. Strengthen them in body, renew their mind, and ignite their spirit. Help them to see that their health is not just about them, but about serving You and others more fully.

Send them out with courage to take their next steps in faith, even when the path ahead feels unclear. Fill them with Your peace when life is overwhelming. Let Your Word be their foundation, Your Spirit be their guide, and Your love be their motivation.

Lord, may they leave this book not just inspired, but committed to walking daily with You—stronger, freer, and ready to serve.

In the powerful name of Jesus, Amen.

For up-to-date resources: **TheBodyBuildingPotter.com**

To book Coach Cathleen for a speaking engagement, please email her manager Denae at *Denae@UnderTheHorizon.net*.

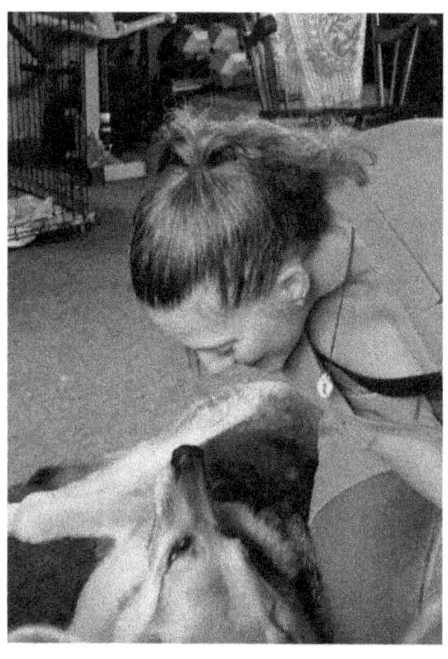

If you've made it this far, I want you to know my personal, God-centered transformation didn't happen alone. I was surrounded by people who loved me, supported me, and stood with me — especially my amazing family, whose patience and faith carried me more than they know. And I want you to know who Hannah was, whom I dedicated this book to. She was my heart dog — a gift from God who walked with me through the hardest seasons of my life. She loved me without condition, stayed when I was breaking, and quietly carried more of my pain than she ever should have had to.

On the day this book's cover was sent to me, she went home — only after she knew I was okay. Her work was complete, and she could rest. Hannah was there through it all, and her faithfulness is woven into these pages.

www.ingramcontent.com/pod-product-compliance
Lightning Source LLC
Chambersburg PA
CBHW050913260726
48660CB00001B/172